The Skills and Ethics of Professional Touch

"After #MeToo and the COVID pandemic there has been a crisis of touch, especially in professional settings. This well-researched and easily digestible book will help a range of students and professionals navigate this touchy territory. With a wealth of expertise, the authors provide a mixture of scientific explanation, very practical concerns with clients, and provocative theoretical discussion to each chapter, along with helpful features for discussion and reflection. A very readable and informative resource."
—Mark Paterson, Professor of Sociology, *University of Pittsburgh*, USA, and author of *The Senses of Touch: Haptics, Affects and Technologies*

Taina Kinnunen • Jaana Parviainen
Annu Haho

The Skills and Ethics of Professional Touch

From Theory to Practice

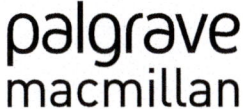

Taina Kinnunen
University of Oulu
Oulu, Finland

Jaana Parviainen
Tampere University
Tampere, Finland

Annu Haho
Laurea University of Applied Sciences
Espoo, Finland

ISBN 978-981-99-4869-7   ISBN 978-981-99-4870-3 (eBook)
https://doi.org/10.1007/978-981-99-4870-3

© The Editor(s) (if applicable) and The Author(s), under exclusive licence to Springer Nature Singapore Pte Ltd. 2023

This work is subject to copyright. All rights are solely and exclusively licensed by the Publisher, whether the whole or part of the material is concerned, specifically the rights of translation, reprinting, reuse of illustrations, recitation, broadcasting, reproduction on microfilms or in any other physical way, and transmission or information storage and retrieval, electronic adaptation, computer software, or by similar or dissimilar methodology now known or hereafter developed.

The use of general descriptive names, registered names, trademarks, service marks, etc. in this publication does not imply, even in the absence of a specific statement, that such names are exempt from the relevant protective laws and regulations and therefore free for general use.

The publisher, the authors, and the editors are safe to assume that the advice and information in this book are believed to be true and accurate at the date of publication. Neither the publisher nor the authors or the editors give a warranty, expressed or implied, with respect to the material contained herein or for any errors or omissions that may have been made. The publisher remains neutral with regard to jurisdictional claims in published maps and institutional affiliations.

Cover credit: lunamarina

This Palgrave Macmillan imprint is published by the registered company Springer Nature Singapore Pte Ltd.
The registered company address is: 152 Beach Road, #21-01/04 Gateway East, Singapore 189721, Singapore

Paper in this product is recyclable.

Acknowledgements

Although we did not know it at the time, the long and multifaceted process that ultimately led to this book started in the late 2000s. Between 2009 and 2011, Jaana Parviainen and Taina Kinnunen co-conducted the research project *New working body: Control and capital*, during which they interviewed secondary schoolteachers, fitness instructors and other professionals in order to investigate new forms of 'body work'. Soon afterwards, another project—*The working body in the post-industrial economy: Professional learning, skills and emotional-aesthetic control* (2011–2014)—provided more nuanced knowledge about various professionals' embodied working skills. Annu Haho conducted her own research project, *Existential suffering of cancer patients in palliative care*, in 2015.

Taina Kinnunen's research on the sense of touch started in the early 2010s when she gathered touch biographies from Finnish people, including client work professionals. Step by step, we authors started to understand the role of touch in different types of body work. We then launched the research project *Professional touch as part of the skills and ethics of elderly care* (2016–2018), in which all of us were involved. This project produced a textbook on professional touch in Finnish (Kinnunen et al. 2019). That book is the basis for this one.

We are grateful to the Finnish Work Environment Fund and the Academy of Finland for funding our research projects. We offer our respectful thanks to the four anonymous reviewers who provided invaluable comments on our book proposal, and to the reviewer of the final manuscript: your suggestions greatly improved our original manuscript. We warmly thank all our academic colleagues and co-researchers who have helped us to develop our ideas about touch over the years. Although it is impossible to name you all, we specifically want to thank Mari Jolkkonen, Johanna Aromaa (Seppänen), Marjo Kolehmainen, Virve Keränen, Eila Estola, Anna-Maija Puroila, Piritta Nätynki, Mari Kangasniemi, Liisa Tainio, Pirkko Tolmunen and Anna Jussilainen.

We also thank all the other colleagues who have given expert comments on our papers on touch in various contexts. We have been blessed to have so many inspiring collaborators from different professional fields, with whom we have discussed and organised diverse projects on touch. We send our heartfelt hugs to you all—especially Eino Saari, Ville Erola, Eija Huttunen and Sanna Tuovinen. We truly thank all the managers and gatekeepers who have given us opportunities to share our interest in touch and learn ever more from real professionals. We are endlessly indebted to all the interviewees and authors who have shared their experiences, views and stories with us. Without your contributions, this book would never have been written. Finally, we wish to express our deepest thanks to Dr. Merl Fluin, whose brilliant proofreading and editing expertise was crucially important during the finalisation of the manuscript, as well as our warm thanks to Dr. Paul Day for his invaluable help with the text.

Contents

1	**Introduction: Touch as a Professional Skill and Ethical Stance**	1
	1.1 An Essential But Unseen Work Tool	1
	1.2 A Timely Issue: From COVID-19 to #MeToo	5
	1.3 Touch as Body Work	8
	1.4 Human Beings Are Hardwired to Touch	13
	1.5 Learning to Touch in a Professional Manner: What Does It Mean?	17
	1.6 How to Read This Book	22
	References	24
2	**Touch as a Professional Skill**	29
	2.1 Mapping Multidimensional Functions of Professional Touch	30
	2.1.1 Connecting Touch	33
	2.1.2 Procedural Touch	35
	2.1.3 Assisting and Guiding Touch	38
	2.1.4 Exploratory Touch	41
	2.1.5 Caring and Comforting Touch	42
	2.1.6 Therapeutic Touch	45
	2.1.7 Protective and Controlling Touch	46
	2.2 Merging Functions of Touch	47
	2.3 Multisensory Messages	50
	2.4 Styles and Techniques of Professional Touch	52
	2.5 Managing one's Own Affects and Emotions	58
	2.6 Listening to the Client	61
	2.7 Thematic Learning Tasks	64
	2.7.1 Reflection Activities	64
	2.7.2 Fieldwork	65
	2.7.3 Case Study	65
	References	66
3	**Socialisation into Touch Cultures**	71
	3.1 Primary Socialisation into Touch	72
	3.2 Culture-Bound Touch	78
	3.3 Varied Skinscapes	85

3.4	Gendered and Sexualised Professional Touch	90
3.5	Complex Touch Cultures: How Do I Survive?	96
3.6	Thematic Learning Tasks	101
	3.6.1 Reflection Activities	101
	3.6.2 Fieldwork	102
	3.6.3 Case Study	102
References		103

4 Technology-Mediated Touch ... 107
4.1	Digital Connection Is the Oxygen We Breathe	108
4.2	Work Digitalisation	109
4.3	Digital Proxemics: Information Technology (Dis)connecting People at Work	112
4.4	Touching with and Through Technological Tools	116
4.5	Triadic Touch: Technologies as Actors in Client Interactions	120
4.6	Work Automation, Cyborgs and Robotic Touch	124
4.7	Material Touching: When Artefacts Touch You	129
4.8	Touch Deprivation in Digitised Working Environments?	131
4.9	Thematic Learning Tasks	134
	4.9.1 Reflection Activities	134
	4.9.2 Fieldwork	137
	4.9.3 Case Study	137
References		138

5 The Ethics of Professional Touch ... 143
5.1	Touching as an Ethical Dilemma for Professionals	144
5.2	Normative Ethics and Touch	145
5.3	Descriptive Ethics of Touch in an Organisational Context	148
5.4	Facing the Other and Embodied Ethics	151
5.5	Presence, Sensitivity and Empathy	155
5.6	Dignity and Value Awareness with Vulnerable People	160
5.7	Ethics of Non-touch Policies	163
5.8	Rewarding Touch Intertwined with Professional Identity	165
5.9	Moral Distress	168
5.10	Thematic Learning Tasks	173
	5.10.1 Reflection Activities	173
	5.10.2 Fieldwork	174
	5.10.3 Case Study	175
References		175

6 Conclusion: Scenarios and Curriculums of Professional Touch ... 181
6.1	Professional Touch in a Nutshell	181
6.2	Alternative Scenarios for the Future of Professional Touch	182
6.3	Should Touch Skills Be Added to Organisational Mission Statements and Educational Curriculums?	187
References		190

7	**Research Material**...	191
	7.1	Quoted Interviews.....................................	191
	7.2	Archive Materials	192

Index 193

List of Boxes

Box 2.1	Rapid Touch in Customer Service	33
Box 2.2	Tactile Tactics in Business	33
Box 2.3	Lifting Patients Using the Kinaesthetics Method	39
Box 2.4	Making a First Impression Through Bodily Gestures	50
Box 2.5	Hapteces and Haptemes	53
Box 3.1	Culture and Personality	74
Box 3.2	Cultural Sensitivity (Slightly Modified from the Guidelines by the Finnish Institute for Health and Welfare, 2021)	84
Box 3.3	Changes in European Skinscape	87
Box 3.4	Varied Sensory Orders	89
Box 4.1	Maurice Merleau-Ponty's Phenomenological Formulation of the Body	112
Box 4.2	Don Ihde's Four Basic Forms of Technological Mediation	119
Box 4.3	Cannulisation as an Example of a Triadic Relationship	121
Box 4.4	Three approaches to ethics in care robotics	128
Box 5.1	Touching from the Perspective of Beauchamp and Childress' Bioethical Principles	147
Box 5.2	Dignity Materialised as Presence and Touching Between Practical Nurses and Elderly People in End-of-Life Care	161
Box 5.3	A Boisterous Child in a Day Care Group	170
Box 5.4	A Violent Dementia Patient in Long-Term Residential Care	171
Box 6.1	Skills and Ethics of Touch Required from Individual Employees and Organisations	188
Box 6.2	Content and Goals of Touch Education	189

List of Tables

Table 4.1 Summary of key concepts related to technology-mediated touch 135
Table 5.1 How theories of normative ethics align with professionals' questions about touch practices 148
Table 6.1 Prerequisites for the realisation of a positive touch scenario 186

1

Introduction: Touch as a Professional Skill and Ethical Stance

Abstract

Touch dominates our everyday lives, but it is surprising that it has only recently become the subject of research. In several occupations, touch is an instrumental, assistive or emotional tool for making a connection with the client, performing necessary procedures and generating positive psychophysical outcomes. This chapter foregrounds fundamental criteria for professional touch as a working skill and considers how touch embodies professional ethics. It introduces the conceptual framework, empirical material and theoretical underpinnings that frame the book. This chapter provides a brief overview of touch as an essential but unseen work tool and explores touch as a timely issue from COVID-19 to #metoo campaign. We introduce the key concepts of 'body work' and 'emotional work', and findings of recent neuroscientific research on touch. The chapter gives guidelines for understanding 'professional touch' as professional know-how and embodied ethics.

1.1 An Essential But Unseen Work Tool

It is morning. Sara, who works in home care as a practical nurse, comes to Mary's home to help her with her morning tasks. Mary is an elderly person who lives alone in a flat in the suburbs. Sara wishes her good morning from the flat's entrance hall, takes off her coat and comes into Mary's bedroom. Mary is already awake but still in bed. After asking how Mary's night has been, Sara helps her to pull down the blanket, turn to one side and place her lower legs outside the bed. Mary is now sitting on the edge of the bed. Next, Sara supports her at the armpits and knees so that she can stand up and grab hold of her walking frame. After making sure that Mary is not feeling dizzy, Sara assists her to walk to the bathroom by walking alongside her, accompanying Mary's movements with her entire body. Sara is constantly ready to react should Mary stumble.

In the bathroom, Mary takes off her pyjama bottoms and sits on the toilet. Sara puts on some gloves, detaches a transdermal patch from Mary's back, wipes her back and affixes a new patch. Before removing her gloves, Sara also assists Mary with her intimate hygiene and changes her clothes and incontinence briefs. She encourages Mary to wash her face and hands and helps her to brush her hair. Next, Mary and Sara move to the kitchen, where Sara prepares porridge for Mary, who sits at the table. When she serves the porridge, Sara wishes Mary bon appétit by patting her on the shoulder. She also puts Mary's morning pills in Mary's hand and makes sure she is able to swallow them. While Mary is eating, Sara records her morning visit on a smartphone app. Mary reads a newspaper as she eats, while Sara prepares to visit another client. Before Sara leaves, she strokes Mary's hand and wishes her a nice day.

Sara's morning visit to Mary's home is an imaginary example of a typical daily encounter between a practical nurse and a home care client. The description is based on a co-researcher's experiences as a nurse and her observations of her colleagues' work routines in home care. The description illustrates how integral touch is to care work, as both a work skill and an ethical stance. Touch fulfils various functions, ranging from creating a connection with the client and assisting them to conduct everyday activities to performing care procedures. Further, touch is an effective means of comforting and encouraging the client and giving them a feeling of safety. The example also illustrates how a smartphone is included in a care worker's normal multitasking.

Touch is often associated exclusively with our most emotionally or sexually intimate relationships, from infancy to adulthood. This is why touching that is 'too free' is often regarded negatively: it 'signifies a closeness of connection that has not been established formally' (Cranny-Francis, 2011, p. 469). In a work context, touch is perceived as a taboo and a potential danger in many sectors and cultural environments (Fuller et al., 2011)—all the more so in pandemic situations (Dawson & Dennis, 2021) and amid the more general politicisation of touch, phenomena to which we return throughout this book. Current discussions, however, often neglect the fact that touch is at the core of many professional tasks.

In a number of occupations, touch is an instrumental, assistive, communicative, emotional and/or therapeutic tool for making a connection with the client, performing necessary procedures and generating positive psychophysical outcomes. Indeed, it is impossible to imagine working in most healthcare and social work professions without touching. Further, touch is essential for early childhood or primary education professionals, physical education instructors, and workers in the beauty and wellness industries. Even the various tasks of police officers, security guards, volunteer workers and caregivers are based on different touches—whether protecting, persuading, encouraging or caring. Both task-oriented and client-oriented touches can be performed in ways that help the client—the fundamental criterion for professional touch—and can be developed as a working skill that embodies professional ethics.

We use the term 'client work' to refer to occupations where professionals interact with clients through touch, either in contact with the skin or via technological devices. Almost all face-to-face client work requires some tactile communication skills—for example, shaking hands with a client, or expressing agreement, empathy, joy or other emotions in certain situations. However, this book focuses on client work that is essentially or primarily performed by touch and where touch is used in multiple ways to carry out necessary work tasks. This includes healthcare (especially nursing), education and social work, fields where our own academic research—conducted over the last 20 years from anthropological, philosophical and scientific nursing perspectives—and professional work experience have revealed the necessity to discuss this topic. In addition, we analyse the use of touch in the work tasks of other professions, particularly beauticians, masseurs, athletics coaches and police officers.

The groundwork for our argument in this book was laid in our earlier research on professional touch (Kinnunen et al., 2019), touch cultures (Kinnunen, 2013; Kinnunen & Kolehmainen, 2019), more-than-human touch (Nätynki et al., 2023), the 'new working body' and affective work (Kinnunen & Parviainen, 2016; Kinnunen & Seppänen, 2009; Parviainen, 2014, 2018; Parviainen & Aromaa, 2017; Parviainen & Kortelainen, 2019), care robotics and the digitalisation of care work (Parviainen et al., 2019; Parviainen & Pirhonen, 2017; Van Aerschot & Parviainen, 2020), and nursing ethics (Haho, 2017, 2020; Puroila & Haho, 2017). For those earlier studies, we collaborated with our students and colleagues Mari Jolkkonen, Arja Sarasoja, Tuija Koivunen and Johanna Aromaa (Seppänen) to interview dozens of professionals. Altogether, we interviewed thirty nurses or practical nurses who worked in various social and healthcare services (home care, hospital wards, sheltered housing, geriatric wards and psychogeriatric wards), one doctor, one sexual therapist, eleven teachers and twelve students of healthcare at two universities of applied sciences, fourteen secondary schoolteachers, two professionals in the beauty and well-being industries, eighteen fitness instructors at health clubs and ten recruitment consultants. Further, we interviewed eight cancer patients in palliative care. We utilise extracts from and analyses of these interviews throughout this book, referring to interviewees by their pseudonyms, nationalities and professions. The cited interviewees are listed at the end of the book (Sect. 7.1).

Naturally, we also provide multiple real-life cases from other studies conducted in different countries and cultures. Further, we utilise research material that consists of 'touch biographies' collected from sixty-eight ordinary Finnish people of different ages and social backgrounds. Touch biographies are written accounts of how the authors were socialised into and experienced touch during their lifetimes, how they touched other humans and non-humans and how they were touched by others. The original idea of collecting these biographies emerged in 2011, when Taina Kinnunen investigated how lived 'skinscapes' (Howes, 2010)—including their natural, material and social elements—vary across generations in Finland. She issued a public call for entries to a writing competition *Touch in Finland—warmth, trust or fear?* (2011–2012) in cooperation with the Folklore Archives of the Finnish Literature Society (FLS). Many of the biographies we cite in this book were either authored by client work professionals or contained interesting reflections on touch from a client's perspective. These biographies provide affectively loaded accounts of diverse experiences that the authors were recalling years or even decades later, and which thus speak to the significance of touch in encounters between professionals and clients. We also utilise some written narratives collected during another public call *The nurse I will never forget* (2000). Both sets of material collected during these projects are archived in the FLS's Traditional and Contemporary Culture Archive in Helsinki, Finland. We therefore refer to these written stories as 'archive research materials' in our list of research materials (Sect. 7.2).

In today's business-oriented jargon, students, patients, children and prisoners are all considered 'clients', and this reflects the wider commercialisation of the healthcare, schooling, education and security sectors (e.g. Hogan et al., 2018; Skountridaki, 2019). We think that the ability to harness one's know-how to meet the client's needs must always be at the heart of client work, whether in the public or private sector. At the same time, however, we argue that the working practices and ethics of healthcare, social work and education in particular should follow logics and practices that extend beyond business management and commercial customer service. The work of a teacher or nurse has a deeper meaning than responding to the student's or patient's immediate wishes in the name of customer satisfaction. Nevertheless, for practical purposes, we use 'client' as a general term, in the same way as we use the term 'professional'. However, when the context is more specific, we also talk about nurses, doctors, patients, teachers and children, for example.

Australian medical instructors state that health professionals use four senses in their daily work routines: sight, hearing, smell and touch. As touching is a 'nuanced, complex and highly context specific behaviour with significant positive potentialities but also dangers, appropriate use of touch is central to effective and compassionate care', as Lorna Davin et al. (2019) argue. However, touch has barely been addressed in the training and education of healthcare professionals. Students of nursing mostly learn about necessary touch in the context of performing procedures, while medical and dental students learn to use touch for exploratory purposes. Until the COVID-19 pandemic brought about the strict regulation of tactile contact, touch was an unseen aspect not just of client work but of everyday life, and people did not think about it much.

Indeed, in many jobs in client work, touch blends into the routines so seamlessly that it is almost impossible to identify it as a specific communication or working tool. For example, the body and touch have traditionally been understood as the heart of nursing practice on one hand, but they have been 'strangely absent' from nursing theory on the other (Draper, 2015). Further, the emergence of new medical technologies is constantly eroding the role of touch in nursing practice, although touch nevertheless remains present, albeit in transformed forms. Studies have shown that when nurses and preschool teachers start thinking about the role of touch in their work, they are often surprised to discover how pervasive it actually is. For instance, Madeline Gleeson and Agnes Higgins (2009), who interviewed psychiatric nurses in Ireland, found that nurses were surprised at how frequently they used touch in their work without being conscious of it, even though they had internalised psychiatry's 'taboo' against it and tried to use touch in a strictly regulated manner. Our own interviews with nurses revealed that 'professional touch' was often associated only with affective communication or therapeutic touch, a kind of 'extra' touch in addition to the necessary procedures. On the other hand, when we asked about the role of touch in their work, there were some interviewees who replied that nursing *was* touching: 'Touch, that's what my work is all about!', as 'Emma', a student who was specialising in gerontology and medical-surgical nursing put it.

We agree with Emma. Touch is inherent to all working practices in nursing, from necessary care practices and medical procedures to everyday communication and the generation of positive affective states in the client. If touch constitutes the 'silent culture of nursing' (Van Dongen & Elema, 2001, p. 150), it is little wonder that professionals whose work involves something other than direct care for the client's body seldom associate their working routines with touch. For example, few police officers consider themselves to be professionals of touch. However, as we propose, the identification of the various ways in which touch is used as a tool in client work can benefit police officers and security guards too. It can help them not only to grasp the specific nature of their work, but also to understand how specific styles of touch contribute to their professional identity and public role. Further, any tactile contact with a client causes a psychophysical reaction in the professional's body too. Therefore, understanding touch as a multidimensional part of working practices can help professionals to cope with their workload while simultaneously strengthening the rewarding aspects of their work.

1.2 A Timely Issue: From COVID-19 to #MeToo

Touch is a topic that permeates several contemporary phenomena. At the time of writing, the global pandemic has shattered fundamental societal structures and practices, in some cases irreversibly so. According to the World Health Organization's (WHO) general guidelines, everyone should avoid touch whenever possible and maintain a safe physical distance from others. The lurking danger of infection has changed client work encounters, especially face-to-face interactions, in dramatic ways. Novel touch constellations and forms of intimacy have emerged, while previous 'good' ways of touching, such as when relatives or healthcare staff are comforting the dying, have been hindered (Driessen et al., 2021; Green & Moran, 2021). No one knows yet what kind of communal trauma these decisions have wrought, or how deep that trauma runs. Nevertheless, all kinds of touch were reduced to the minimum if not forbidden, and workers were (and are) expected to use the necessary protective gear. The WHO (2022) points out that while 'health workers are central to the COVID-19 pandemic response', they also 'face higher risks of infection in their efforts to protect the greater community and are exposed to hazards such as psychological distress, fatigue and stigma'. Other client work professionals who work in close physical contact with their clients or colleagues face the same problems to some extent, although their role in the struggle against the pandemic has been less critical.

One concern about the long-term outcomes of COVID-19 policies is that they will have serious impacts on client work and touch cultures in general. There is the danger of a demonisation of touch that may lead in future to the unwarranted avoidance of touch and the overuse of gloves in healthcare, for example. Even before the pandemic, nurses reported that they wore gloves (for their own protection) during every patient contact, even though global and national guidelines emphasise the importance of distinguishing between the necessary and unnecessary use of gloves (Anedda et al., 2020; Nazarko, 2020). Another potential negative consequence of the strict regulation of touch is that clients may be forced to use digitalised services only, or to accept cuts to services. None of these future prospects appear to be ethically tenable outcomes of the pandemic, despite the benefits of strict touch regulation policies (Nist et al., 2020; Roberts, 2020). With regard to digitalised services, even before the outbreak of the pandemic, there was growing anxiety about the loss of human touch due to the accelerated digitalisation of everyday life, including in client work (e.g. Gross, 2019). Many of us feel that even though we spend hours every day writing emails, chatting on Facebook or checking our 'likes' on X, something is missing. We feel lonely.

It is widely reported that economically justified staffing reductions, or simple recruitment difficulties, have made it difficult to carry out all the necessary tasks in healthcare, social work and various levels of education. In many countries, for example, the average time spent per client on different forms of elderly care has fallen, and maltreatment scandals have become all too familiar. Elder abuse is a worldwide problem: two out of three elderly care professionals in different countries had witnessed it in their workplaces before the COVID-19 pandemic (Yon et al., 2017), and it is estimated that the rate nearly doubled after the outbreak of the pandemic (Chang & Levy, 2021). The term 'abuse' refers to acts (or a lack of appropriate action) that may be perceived as violence causing physical, sexual, psychological or emotional damage to the abused person. Sometimes elder abuse takes the form of serious neglect and a deep violation of human dignity. Many strategies have been implemented worldwide, including the WHO's global strategy to prevent abuse, and some interventions have proven to be successful.

Characteristically, wealthy countries that struggle with the challenge of arranging elderly care tend to fantasise about solving the problem with smart houses, care robots and new digital applications. Technology has probably enhanced many processes in client work, including elderly care, and many individuals find online services helpful and convenient. However, it is difficult to imagine that a society where digital devices, information systems and robots have largely replaced body-to-body encounters will be ideal for the majority of people. In reality, professionals are usually expected to soften the presence and touch of technical devices. Chapter 4 is dedicated to multifaceted questions about the relationship between technology and embodied, tactile client work, including questions about the automatisation of client encounters, technostress, gathering-around technologies, technology-mediated touch and robotic touch.

Instead of replacing human touch with technologies, might the systematic inclusion of touch in technological intervention strategies help to develop new solutions to resourcing problems, and therefore become a topic of communication skills training? One symptom of the failure to provide reasonable resources and arrangements for care is the growing conflict and tension between professionals and clients, which has been reported in several countries (Edward et al., 2014; Uno, 2021; Van Keer et al., 2015). For instance, patients' aggression towards and sexual harassment of nurses and other healthcare staff has increased in recent years (Kahsay et al., 2020). An explanation for this may be the increased number of people with memory impairments. However, miscommunication has also been identified as a potential trigger for incidents (Wilk et al., 2018). Research findings indicate that a professional's communication style greatly impacts on the nature of their encounters with clients. As we will discuss throughout the book, managing to use touch in productive ways in different situations can sometimes be crucially important for successful client encounters.

Further, touch implicitly lies at the heart of many of today's most heated queer and feminist debates, from the #metoo movement to the politics of safe spaces. Touching has become an exceedingly politicised act through which intersectional power relations are actualised in multiple ways. Touch is gendered everywhere in culturally specific ways, and it is intertwined with demands for equality. Phenomena such as activism around consent, debates over breastfeeding and various legislative bans on homosexual contact in many countries all converge on the gendered politics of touch—even though these debates seldom analyse touch explicitly (Kinnunen & Kolehmainen, 2019). In addition, the growing awareness and fear of child abuse, especially in Anglo-American countries, has led to a situation where male workers in particular are instructed not to touch children under any circumstances (Sect. 3.4). Our own interviews with Finnish secondary school teachers revealed that male teachers categorically chose not to touch their male students on any occasion, whereas they might hug female students on presenting them with their school graduation certificates, if they had sought and obtained permission beforehand.

Would it be best, then, for a male teacher, doctor, nurse or youth leader to refrain from touch of any kind, in order to avoid accusations of sexual harassment? Our answer is no. To do so would be to throw the baby out with the bathwater. The categorical avoidance of touch is not the way to root out violating touch. Respecting the client's personal space should not be equated with refraining from touch. Quite the opposite is needed: a cherishing touch that appreciates and cares. We believe that a caring touch and a harming touch differ so starkly from each other that it is not plausible to refrain from touch on the grounds that a client might confuse one for the other. Nevertheless, it must be acknowledged that two different people may not speak the same tactile language and may therefore, at least momentarily, misinterpret each other. However, it is probable that clients often expect and want to be touched by professionals, more so than we believe, especially when they are in a vulnerable state. Touch deprivation is a real issue, and it is possible to imagine alternative scenarios where touch will undergo a renaissance and more multiple uses will be made of it in client work than ever before. Lockdowns and the regulation of client work practices have pushed many of us to fully realise that touch is a fundamental human way of being with others, a basic need without which it is hard to live a meaningful life.

After all, despite the most innovative forms of substitution, numerous client work tasks are still almost impossible to perform without touch. Assisting patients with severe diseases or impairments in different care settings, comforting children in day care or at school, protecting clients from damaging themselves during policing tasks—all of these simply cannot be performed without touching the client. Therefore, the mission of this book is not only to bring touch and embodiment back into the core of client work (cf. Draper, 2015), but also to scrutinise its potential to resolve current problems. Nevertheless, we acknowledge that touch is a conflicted practice, and there is an urgent need to discuss insensitive, violent or rough touch in professional practices, as well as the unwanted touching that professionals themselves experience (see also Davin et al., 2019; Kelly et al., 2017).

1.3 Touch as Body Work

Thinking about client work from the perspective of touch brings the embodiment of work into focus. The practices and bodies involved need to be addressed from different perspectives of *body work* to understand the multilayered workings of touch. 'Body work' or 'body labour' is a concept that has been discussed widely in sociological and cultural body research (e.g. Gimlin, 2007; Twigg, 2006; Wolkowitz, 2006) and organisation studies (e.g. Hassard et al., 2000; Rajan-Rankin, 2018; Witz et al., 2003). Much of this discussion encompasses professions in healthcare, social work, sports instruction, and the beauty and wellness industries and aims to make the presence, practices and relations of bodies visible in these professions (e.g. García-Santesmases et al., 2022; Lanoix, 2013; Parviainen, 2014, 2018; Parviainen & Kortelainen, 2019; Sunanta, 2020; Twigg et al., 2011; Wolf et al., 2022). There are some variations in the meanings of the concept of body work, depending on the form of body work under discussion. These include understanding the body work as (1) paid labour carried out directly on the bodies of others, (2) 'emotional' or 'affective labour', i.e. management of one's own and others' emotions/affects, (3) the work performed on one's own working body and the management of its performances and (4) the production of bodies through work (Gimlin, 2007; Twigg et al., 2011).

In this book, we consider touch as a fundamental part especially of the first two of these forms of body work, although they in any case extend to and overlap with the latter forms too. The first form is naturally the most essential when thinking about touch as a working practice, since this conceptualising of body work refers to 'direct, hands-on activities on other bodies, such as assessing, diagnosing, handling, treating, manipulating, and monitoring bodies' (Twigg et al., 2011). In other words, the client's body is an object to be treated, 'a site of labour' (Van Dongen & Elema, 2001, p. 151), in this form of body work. The work of beauticians, masseurs, (practical) nurses and physiotherapists are all examples of 'pure' body work, as Jan Draper (2015, p. 2237) illustrates in the case of nursing:

> [Body work] involves observing bodies; learning to 'read' them by searching skilfully for outward signs of inner goings on; cleaning and bathing bodies; medicating bodies; touching bodies; preserving body boundaries and employing great care to prevent and manage leakage and yet, conversely, sometimes purposefully breaking body boundaries to insert enemas, injections or nasogastric tubes; alleviating pain and then sometimes, of necessity,

inflicting it; and then, a most powerful example of body-work, the laying out of the dead body.

As Draper reveals, a nurse's body work consists of performing necessary care tasks and procedures on the client's body by touching it with hands or medical instruments. In nursing science this kind of touching is referred to as 'procedural', 'necessary' or 'instrumental' touch, and we consider it in Sect. 2.1.2 as one of the main functions of professional touch. When degree programmes in fields such as nursing, sports science and dentistry address touch, the discussion generally concerns touch. Students are given guidance on how to enter the client's personal space correctly when carrying out procedural procedures. The basic rule is that the client should always be warned before being touched by hand or with an instrument. In extreme cases, procedural touch applies to situations where the worker reduces physical contact with the client to the absolute minimum. This is typical in dentistry and other procedure-dominated medical work.

Although the research literature referenced here focuses mainly on nursing, we extend the discussion to other professions and various types of necessary touch. A police officer who manoeuvres an arrested person into a police car, or a paramedic who transports an injured patient from the ambulance to the operating theatre, also uses touch predominantly for instrumental purposes. Assistive touch is also a typical form of necessary touching used to help a disabled client or small child perform certain tasks independently (e.g. García-Santesmases et al., 2022). Healthcare professionals often also use investigative touch to obtain information about a patient's bodily condition, as do beauticians and masseurs with their clients. Throughout this book, we will address various aspects that need to be considered in the context of necessary touch to ensure the success of the procedure and the client's and professional's safety and comfort.

However, in client work, hands-on working through touch is about much more than the performance of necessary procedures or actions. Nursing includes perhaps the widest variety of the functions of touch. In their study of hospital nurses' body work, Zane R. Wolf and colleagues (2022) identified a total of 128 typical nursing interventions that nurses carry out on patients' bodies using direct or instrument/technology-mediated touch. These items were divided into work task clusters which included Technologic Device Management, Intubation Management, Physical Comfort Facilitation, Mobility Management, Skin/Wound Management, Safety Management, Nutrition Management, Thermoregulation Management, Self-care Facilitation, Respiratory Management, Elimination Management, Electrolyte and Acid/Base Management, Medication Management, Tissue Perfusion Management, Neurologic Management, Assessment Management, Psychological Comfort Promotion, Energy Conservation Management and After Death Care Management.

As this extensive list just of clusters of body work indicates, a great deal of the nurse's body work obviously concerns our second form, 'emotional' and/or 'affective' body work, which brings us to the 'social' and 'expressive' functions of touch. We address these functions predominantly in the context of caring and comforting touch (Sect. 2.1.5), but want to stress that all working through touch is emotional and affective work—the meanings of which overlap but which we are not identical in all contexts. 'Emotional work' is best known from Arlie Hochschild's (1983) legendary work on workers' emotion management. In her best-known empirical case, on the work of flight attendants, she illustrates how inducing or suppressing one's own feelings and creating certain emotional states in clients (like calmness in airline passengers) has become an essential part of client work. Employees are expected to follow 'feeling rules' that comply with the employer's requirements. It is not enough for flight attendants only to give an appearance ('surface acting') of loving their job (and their clients), they must really try to love them ('deep acting'), in the manner in which the employer systematically trains them.

Hochschild's inferences have been tremendously inspiring for body work research, including ours, although we see a greater complexity to emotional work through touch thanks to its demands and multidirectional effects. We agree with Monique Lanoix (2013, p. 95) that care work is 'thickly embodied' *because* of touch, and it is therefore also thickly emotional and affective labour. As Lanoix (ibid., p. 94; see also 2019) states, both caregivers and those receiving care (and their loved ones) expect that 'care should be caring', which separates a human caregiver from a care robot. Even the most basic care routines should ideally be performed by delicate touch, as we stress in Sect. 2.1.2. The emotional and affective aspects of touch are naturally not reduced to nursing but apply also to social workers, childhood educators, teachers, coaches and security experts, although in different ways. A police officer or a guard is expected to convey other emotional messages and create other affective states in their clients than a nurse or a teacher—a point for which Hochschild (1983) provides another reminder by referring to the work of debt collectors. However, both a police officer and a nurse may use protective or distancing touch among other distancing techniques, such as a generally dismissive bodily demeanour and the wearing of uniforms or plastic gloves (Gimlin, 2007, p. 358–360). The function of controlling or protective touch is to protect the client, the professional themselves and bystanders.

We use the terms 'emotion' and 'emotional work' when we address conscious, named and at least partly controllable emotions that individual workers feel and intentionally seek to convey to clients. However, emotional labour cannot just be reduced to its intended emotional expressions and effects. Therefore, we usually use the terms 'affect' and 'affective work', since we take 'affect' as an umbrella term which includes various emotions, sensations, feelings and reactions that are not always easy to name or control but are embodied and registered. The concept of affect better catches the idea of being mutually affected in the act of touch, sometimes in unpredictable and reluctant ways (Kinnunen & Kolehmainen, 2019). 'Affective work' then, better than 'emotional work', conveys the constitutive power of embodied emotions, sensations, feelings and energies that transmit *across* bodies. It directs the attention to 'what affects can do' instead of 'what affects are' (cf. Weeks, 2007, p. 241) and highlights affects as being what *emerges* between the encountering bodies in/through touch, as well as in responses to touch. Some researchers have described both touch and affect as opening or being exposed to the other in undefined and partly unpredictable ways (Irigaray, 1984; Kinnunen &

Kolehmainen, 2019; Manning, 2007; Paterson, 2007). More than 'emotion', 'affect' relates to the understanding of skin as 'porous' and relational, rather than an envelope that separates an individual body from other bodies (Paterson, 2007). Further, we recognise that technological devices and other material objects are often involved in affects and tensions between professionals and clients, and the professional must learn to cope with this (Chap. 4).

The insight of 'relational skins' (Lafrance, 2018) permeates all our addressed themes, since touching is never a one-way or top-down interaction. We emphasise the reciprocity of touch: one cannot touch another without simultaneously being touched oneself. There is no touch without affects. All touches are 'expressive'; they convey emotional signals and transmit affective energies, even unintentionally. The simplest procedural or assistive touch can be performed in several ways; and the client recognises different styles of touch carrying different affective atmospheres and ethical stances towards them (Sect. 2.4). Therefore, although it is important for client work professionals to identify the versatile modes and functions of touch, we stress that, in practical work, the functions intersect and can fulfil the manifold needs of the client. For example, the therapeutic touch refers to massage or other standardised body treatment methods and, in this sense, represents procedural touch, hands-on body work. On the other hand, these techniques strongly aim to influence the client's overall well-being by generating positive affective responses—and clients themselves expect exactly this outcome. It is unnecessary or even impossible to categorise therapeutic touch as either instrumental or expressive touch, and as a form of body work it carries the same ambiguity.

Thinking through relationality about touch and affect means paying attention to the processual nature of touch and its psychophysical happenings in specific situations, which we valorise by citing various empirical research materials, both our own and other researchers'. These materials shed particular light on the different reflections of both client work professionals and clients on their experiences and thoughts about touch, as well as numerous researchers' observations and research results. Although the worker's intentional touch is professional and often routine, it nevertheless generates an embodied affective reaction not only in the client but in the worker, too. At best, touch empowers the worker; at worst, it causes stress and exhaustion. We consider both scenarios in Sect. 3.2, where we analyse how personal lifelong experiences of touch and culturally learnt habits necessarily resonate in the style and experiences of professional touch. Sections 5.8 and 5.9 cover questions of different affects and feelings related to touch, and their connections with professional identity.

We stress that the professional's own experiences of touching and being touched affect how they consciously and unconsciously experience touch as a professional skill and resource. One individual may perceive touch as a natural and rewarding part of their work, whereas for another it may be a burden that they avoid as much as possible. However, their employer's organisational working culture has a great influence on individual workers' touch practices and other ways of communicating with clients, even though the internalisation of those working cultures may not be fully conscious or openly discussed within the organisation community. Here we take a more optimistic approach than Hochschild, who perceives the organisation's feeling rules as problematic from the perspective of employees. She proposed that emotional work leads to the employees' alienation of their inner selves and bodily demeanour. We stress that in an ideal case the feeling rules are supportive but loose enough to give space for individual situational behaviours and embodied ethics based on the multidimensional contextual knowledge and decision-making of the professional. Therefore, this book will advance the notion of 'organised emotional/affective work', which offers a more supportive alternative to professional sensory practices than the restrictive rules of organisational management (cf. Lopez, 2006). Managing touch practices through conscious communal negotiation can be combined with deepening self-knowledge, which not only helps attune to the client's needs but protects the professional civil self in potentially burdening situations. In this sense we see that the organised emotional/affective work extends also to the third form of body work: managing one's own working body's performances through skilful and sensitive communicative acts which may also intentionally or unintentionally brand the organisation.

The fourth form of body work, the production of bodies through work, will be considered throughout the book from different viewpoints. As already mentioned, we address the reciprocal consequences of touch practices which, together with general working conditions, 'produce' the working bodies in several ways by deploying social, timely and material resources and thereby generating affective resonances in working bodies. We further emphasise that although touch practices and related affects are situational, they do not lack cultural or historical continuity. Rather, touching manners, affects—and, perhaps, emotions related to touch even more than affects—are socially learnt and understandable in their cultural contexts. Both sides carry their lived pasts into a tactile encounter. Furthermore, although drawing on the framework of 'body work' leads to focusing on embodied proximities between professionals and clients, it is important to recognise that body work is always shaped by wider social and economic forces and demographic trends, as Julia Twigg and colleagues (2011) stress. Using the example of nursing work and wellness services, they propose that many global phenomena, such as the nationalised and racialised division of care work and beauty services and the related 'high-touch' tourism and migration of providers of body work, have greatly influenced the organisation of body work. Along with these spatial, economic and societal factors, we focus on cultural habits and ideologies that shape and regulate general, and thereby professional, touch practices and their meaning-making.

In any act of touching, it matters who is touching and being touched, and how, when, why, where (see e.g. Saarinen et al., 2021) and in connection with what other sensory gestures this touching takes place, as we stress in Sects. 2.3. and 3.5. The ways we touch and the meanings we attach to touch depend on our socialisation process in a specific sociocultural environment. Body work is never conducted in a social and cultural vacuum. To some extent, we internalise the normative touching patterns not only of our family of origin, but also of our class, gender, age, sexual orientation, and ethnic or religious background, although no one's touching style can be reduced to any single one of these attributes. How professionals and clients touch each other and respond to touch thus depends on cultural learning. Therefore, we will introduce some observed cultural differences between 'low-intensity' and 'high-intensity' touch cultures (Sect. 3.2) and gendered touch norms (Sect. 3.4), which will provide a general framework for the adaptation of touch to multicultural client work environments. The viewpoint is relevant since connecting or 'social' touch through greeting, for example, is the most common form of touch in mundane encounters and may be included as a part of affective body work too. Depending on their culture, people shake hands, exchange kisses on the cheek, rub noses or embrace to mark the beginning or end of an encounter. Although cultural greetings cannot necessarily be directly applied in client encounters, connecting touch is often a natural way to create a rapport with the client and make them feel noticed and respected (Sect. 2.1.1).

One's cultural background is a multifaceted composite. Over the course of one's life, one persists with early habits and adopts new ones. In globalised everyday life, and increasingly pluralistic, multiprofessional and multicultural working environments, it is important to attune oneself to the different sociocultural factors that matter in communication. However, socialisation into touch is a lifelong process. Diverse social networks, education practices and working cultures constantly shape our touch behaviours and resonate in our experiences of touch. We emphasise that a tactile encounter is not simply an event where an individual professional tries to accommodate their own socioculturally 'predetermined' touching style to that of the client. Rather, although one cannot discount one's own background, each encounter offers an opportunity to affect and be affected upon by touch in novel ways, and thus to remould the learnt patterns of touching. Further, each tactile encounter shapes the way the client's and professional's lived histories come to matter in the encounter, thereby providing valuable opportunities for self-reflexion.

1.4 Human Beings Are Hardwired to Touch

> Touch (the right kind, of course) is as powerful and immediate a reward as chocolate or the scent of Mother to an infant. Touch is a primary color in the color scheme of pleasure, wired deep into our nervous system. (Keltner, 2009, p. 181)

American psychologist David Keltner, cited above, equates the rewarding experience that pleasant touch generates in a human body with calorie-rich ingredients like chocolate. He refers to research which indicates that the orbitofrontal cortex region of the brain processes all basic information, helping humans to navigate their physical and social environment in order to survive. Touch has been called the 'mother of the senses', the earliest to develop in the human embryo and the last to remain in the dying body, which indicates its fundamental character for humans and other primates (e.g. Jablonski, 2006; Montagu, 1971). In the evolution of primates, touch was the most archaic sense, playing a crucial role in grasping and standing on branches, selecting food, using tools and making a fire. Of particular interest in this context is the notion that skin and touch developed as main channels for bonding:

touching with the fingers and lips when in physical proximity, and facial expressions when physically separated, are typical ways of bonding and communication for all primates, while many other mammals mainly nuzzle and lick when touching (Jablonski, 2006, p. 103). Indeed, evolutionary anthropologists and psychologists remind us that touch is the most primal expression of the human body and the 'primary language for compassion, love and gratitude—emotions at the heart of trust and cooperation', as Keltner (2009, p. 178) puts it.

In Western traditions, however, touch has long been considered an insignificant, animalistic, primitive, female and childish sense. The dominance of the visual can be traced back to antiquity: when Plato wrote about the senses, he placed vision above the others, describing it as 'divine' (Classen, 1993; Jütte, 2005). Plato favoured vision and hearing, which he considered the more rational, 'higher senses', over the other, 'lower senses', which he believed were more subjective and bound to bodily reactions (see, e.g. Schellekens, 2009). In a similar manner, Aristotle created a hierarchy of the senses, putting vision first, followed by hearing, smell, taste and touch (Johansen, 1997). In the West, vision has almost always ranked as the highest sense from that point on, through the mediaeval age and up to the present day (Sect. 3.3).

The tactile sense was thus not believed to have much to do with the mental activities of higher cognition until cognitive neuroscientists discovered mirror neurons in the 1990s. The functions of mirror neurons include the mechanism underlying the specific type of synaesthesia where individuals experience somatosensory sensations when they see someone else being touched. Before the popularity of touch screens surprised everyone, engineers and designers showed little interest in exploring the role of touch in digital interactions. The digitalisation of culture and the explosive growth of visual information probably first reduced the motivation for wider touch research. With haptic interfaces, interest in the study of touch perception has exploded, but cognitive science-oriented research has focused primarily on human-machine interactions rather than human-to-human interactions. When Fabian Hutmacher (2019) searched the PsycINFO database for studies referring to visual, auditory, gustatory, olfactory or tactile/haptic memory, he found more studies on visual memory than on the memory of all the other sensory modalities combined. While there were several studies on auditory memory, research on haptic memory was extremely limited.

Given the centrality of touch to the perception system, it is surprising that until recently it has been the subject of so little research. We know that touch dominates our everyday lives simply because it is connected to the skin, the largest organ of the human body, with an area of roughly 1.7 square metres in an adult. Tactile acuity differs between body parts: it is greater in hands and fingertips than in limbs and back, for example. The sense of touch also extends to the interior of the body involving proprioception (a sense of bodily position), kinaesthesia (a sense of bodily movement) and the vestibular system (a sense of balance). The term 'haptic perception' or 'haptic system' refers to a more inclusive conception of touch that incorporates all these (or even more) modalities of touch (Obrador, 2012, p. 50; Paterson, 2007). Opinions differ on whether touch can be perceived as uniquely multisensory because of its physical structure or its functional nature (see Batty, 2015; Fulkerson, 2020; Ratcliffe, 2012).

The tactile sense's modalities and multidimensional connections to the different layers of the brain speak in any case to the fundamental importance of the sense of touch. Many types of receptors in different layers of the skin and elsewhere in the body receive touch stimuli and carry information slowly or quickly to the deep and surface parts of the brain. There is a notably vast area in the brains of humans and other primates for processing a wide variety of tactile sensations. Quickly transmitted receptor information tells us immediately whether we are in danger or safe. Regarding this neurologic function of the sense of touch, the neuroscience had long focused on sensations of pain, temperature, pressure and itch, until C-Tactile fibres (CT afferents or C-touch) were identified in the 1990s by microneurography (Vallbo et al., 1993; see also Gross, 2019). These fibres conduct the skin receptor information more slowly to the brain than the fast-conducting neurons, and the signals they carry target different parts of the brain than neurons, which carry signals for 'discriminative' (avoidant) touch contact or tactile manipulation on environment (Cascio et al., 2019). The CT afferents are found mainly in the hairy skin, and they respond particularly to a gentle, slow, caress-like touch performed with moderate pressure (Löken et al., 2009).

Physiologically, the pleasure produced by tactile sensations is often explained by the hormone oxytocin, which has been described as the body's chemical of love, intimacy and care (Uvnäs Moberg, 2003). It is probable that CT-mediated touch and oxytocin release are physiologically connected so that CT fibres act as mediators of oxytocin in caring and affectionate touch (see Cascio et al., 2019, p. 6). The oxytocin system, for its part, is connected to the wider complex systems of brain opioids, transmitters and hormones which all activate on pleasant touch and are critical for mate selection, parental behaviour and other social actions (Cascio et al., 2019; Uvnäs Moberg, 2003), including communication between strangers (e.g. Field, 2003). In this way, touch is connected to perhaps all essential bodily processes such as heartbeat and blood circulation, as well as the respiratory and nervous systems. It activates the parasympathetic nervous system, the body's internal calming system, promotes rest (i.e. recovery from physical and mental exertion) and generates feelings of security and trust.

For a newborn child, human touch is a basic need, like food, sleep and adequate warmth. A baby cannot even grow without a caring touch, because the release of growth hormones is dependent on touch. Without a protective, supportive and gentle touch that surrounds the entire body, the baby is literally in danger of dying. Animal experiments have shown that a mammal baby gets severely ill or even dies if it lacks close contact with its caregiver (Field, 1995; Keltner, 2009). Crying and afraid, a baby needs to get close to a safe person because it has only a rudimentary ability to calm down on its own. Holding the baby in one's arms is the strongest means to achieve this because it communicates protection and security: 'Now you can calm down because the threat has disappeared'. Through an accepting and calming touch, the child learns to regulate its own feelings and emotions. For example, premature babies have been found to develop faster when they are embraced and held by hand in an incubator (see Field, 2003). Several studies have stressed the importance of sufficient affectionate touch during childhood. Not only is this important for early physiological and psychological development, but it also deeply impacts on personality and intimate relationships in adulthood. Neuroscientists Gallace and Spence (2010, p. 178) state that 'early tactile experiences […] might strongly contribute to shaping and characterising the emotional, relational, cognitive, and neural functioning of the adult individual' (see Sect. 3.1).

Nowadays, the importance of touch for an individual's sense of security, of being bonded to the caregiver, being loved and part of the 'herd', is widely recognised in medicine, psychology, ethology and evolutionary anthropology. Further, there is convincing scientific evidence of the interconnection between exposure to touch, psychophysical health and overall well-being. Caring touch not only activates the body's 'security system', it also blocks the stress-related and other harmful psychophysical processes of the body (e.g. Jakubiak & Feeney, 2017; Uvnäs Moberg, 2003). There is no wonder that, along with the growing awareness of scientific knowledge, interest in activating the parasympathetic nervous system and oxytocin release is manifested in the popularity of various contact therapies, mindfulness techniques or 'free hugs' campaigns. The needier and more vulnerable a person is, the more receptive they are to the messages of touch. For a person who is severely ill, living with dementia, elderly or dying, touch is a crucial connection to the world and its people. For a person who has suffered violence, recently lost a loved one or been traumatised by war, a gentle touch can mean the restoration of faith and the awakening of hope.

Human beings are born with sensory organs, neural systems and brain structures that process tactile impulses and information in a similar way. The functions and practices of touch in professional settings are partly universal. A person who is in pain or dying simply needs to be in proximity to another human, even a client work professional, regardless of social or cultural barriers. For a child, the secure embrace of an adult is vital. Caring touch transmits sympathy and support during the most momentous and frightening moments of a human life. Laying one's hands on someone's shoulder or caressing their forehead are effective ways of expressing compassion and transmitting the message: 'I am here for you, and I accept the way you are'.

Therefore, alongside one's awareness of social and cultural differences, it is important to understand that the meanings and effects of touch extend beyond languages and cultures. Touch may be the most effective way to bring together people from different backgrounds. Since touch is a newborn's first immediate contact with other people and the world, it can be argued that we understand the messages and signals of touch before we understand spoken language. Similarly, for a person in palliative care, touch is their last contact with the world and its meanings, beyond spoken words. The significance of touch in human communication is to be found at the point where mind and body unite. The experience of touch is beyond words, although the nature and effect of touch can be strongly experienced and we therefore strive to capture nuances by talking about warm, cold, hard, light, limp, stiff or soft touch, for example (Sect. 2.4). Touch is to some extent felt as either empowering or incapacitating one's own or the other person's body.

The benefits of the proper use of touch in client work are widely reported. Our own research has also demonstrated that a single caring touch from a professional can be a pivotal experience for a client that they will remember in detail, even decades later. A child growing up in an insecure background can experience a social worker's or a teacher's caring touch as a turning point in their life which may open up a totally new world of emotions. For a lonely person, the gentle touch of a hairdresser can be a high point in their everyday life. Likewise, other kinds of touch (or its avoidance) leave strong memory traces. One worker's rough or careless touch can destroy a client's confidence in the whole profession the worker represents. All in all, touch memories are stored deep in the body, as middle-aged 'Laura' described in her account of experiences as a patient.

> There they go along, good and bad remembrances, in the body's memory. Cool grass, a dog's lick, an arm holding one's arm, stroking one's hair – a simple empathic gaze, a little tiny gesture, a hint of understanding. Also, the pain that was not heard, someone turning their back on you and their mental absence. There they are in your subconscious, in your dreams and body, and they come from there to fix or break, to comfort or haunt. (Laura, Finnish patient)

1.5 Learning to Touch in a Professional Manner: What Does It Mean?

> It is their work and I would not expect that they should or would want to build a deeper relationship; I would not want to impose that on them or him. However, I do want them to care for him, which means that I want their touch to be sympathetic, soft, or even warm. I want them to help him feel comfortable, certainly, but also respected. (Lanoix, 2013, p. 94)

Monique Lanoix aptly captures the core of professionality of touch when describing her expectations of the nurses taking care of her injured husband in a long-term-care residential facility. By 'professional touch', we mean touching with a definite professional consciousness, attitude and ethical intention, where the client's body is touched purposefully, respectfully and sometimes emotionally, but not primarily in a personal or intimate manner (e.g. Benner, 2004; Bottorff, 1993; Bush, 2001; Connor & Howett, 2009). Professionals' abilities and responsibilities to distinguish their civilian selves from their professional roles are therefore important, since they are not supposed—or allowed—to touch their clients in the same way as they touch their family members, such as kissing and caressing a spouse's cheek to say goodnight. Nevertheless, touch at work should be genuine, trusting and respectful in a human and personal way (Draper, 2015; Holopainen et al., 2014). This form of professionalism should be manifested in daily encounters with clients. Professional touch should never be aggressive, abusive or offensive to human dignity.

Further, professional touch is always justified by its context; it involves adjusting its practices and affective aims appropriately to each task and situation. In other words, the right to touch is related to situation-specific work duties and the professional should not touch the client in the same way when off duty. Overall, the right is acquired through one's professional training and terms of employment, whether one works as an employee or is self-employed. In many respects, client work is about building a confident corporeal rapport with the client, which is the focus of this book. It requires an effort to gauge the client's psychophysical condition and respond to their needs in a professionally sound manner. This implies that professional touch and other sensory gestures—speech, silence, tone of voice, gaze, touch—are adjusted to each encounter in its social and cultural contexts (Sects. 2.3 and 3.5). In other words, professionals need situational awareness of the right thing to do at a particular moment. Therefore, the professionalism of touch includes two parallel and interrelated dimensions: (1) the professional ethics of touching, i.e. the ethics of touch, and (2) touch as professional know-how.

Professional ethics frequently include rules, recommendations, standards, regulations and guidelines which various occupational groups are committed and legally expected to follow. Professional ethics is thus to a great extent *normative*, although it includes rather general promises made to clients, societies and humankind more generally. Each profession has its shared international ethical code, although national legislations may vary. For instance, the International Code of Ethics for Nurses states that 'inherent in nursing is respect for human rights, including cultural rights, the rights to life and choice, to dignity and to be treated with respect' (International Council of Nurses, 2021). The international code of police ethics is 'to safeguard lives and property; to protect the innocent against deception, the weak against oppression or intimidation and the peaceful against violence or disorder; and to respect the constitutional rights of all to liberty, equality, and justice' (International Association of Chiefs of Police, 2023). Despite different emphases within each client work profession, there are many internationally shared ethical principles or values, such as human dignity, equality, justice, self-determination and truthfulness. These permeate the professional ethical codes discussed in this book, as we address especially in Sect. 5.2.

Therefore, instead of going through the ethical regulations and specificities of every profession, we discuss the general legislative and ethical principles and conditions that need to be considered in order to fulfil the requirement of respecting universal principles of sustainable professional ethics in the context of touching the clients. Regardless of their value as general human guidelines, we believe that normative ethics usually provide too abstract (or idealised) a framework for practical level action. However, they help the professional to a deeper understanding of the origins of ideas about a good and correct way of touching. On the other hand, professionals must make prompt decisions about touch practices based on their own intuition and judgement, their 'gut feeling', without knowing in that specific situation where their 'ethical feelings' come from. This has inspired us to formulate specific questions concerning rights, responsibilities, virtues, equality and willingness, through which professionals can learn more about classical ethical dilemmas and reflect on their own decision-making, beliefs and working propensities (Table 5.1). A theoretical knowledge of ethics can also help the professional reflect on different situations afterwards, learn from them and develop individual and shared touch practices.

1.5 Learning to Touch in a Professional Manner: What Does It Mean?

We further think that normative ethics needs alongside it a *descriptive ethics* that recognises the messiness of everyday working life. As many real-life cases illustrate, there are situations where the professional is forced to touch the client against their will or without their permission. For a police officer, teacher or nurse, this may happen daily. These professionals need to know the criteria for involuntary but necessary touch, to follow official protocols and their profession's ethical guidelines, duly adjusted for actual circumstances and to report all events carefully. Numerous contextual issues need to be taken into account and one's actions adjusted to them. External societal and environmental circumstances—such as suddenly reduced resources due to natural disaster, war, large-scale accidents or pandemics—make it challenging to provide touch in ethically sustainable ways. Other factors, such as cultural or institutional rules, may also designate who can touch whom (e.g. who is dirty or clean enough to touch or be touched) and even which workers have official permission to touch (or not touch) certain clients. Spontaneous touching may be restricted, and there is a risk that some clients will become marginalised and others privileged.

Therefore, drawing on discussions of relational ethics, we develop a novel approach to *embodied ethics* that provides principles for how professionals can be present with, approach and behave towards clients in fair and ethically sound ways, while also taking account of the many factors that can limit touch interactions. We insist that all touch practices and ethical promises should be based on value awareness, empathy, presence and sensitivity, and be aimed at the client's well-being and benefit, even when the client initially suspects or even resists some practices (Fredriksson, 1999; Holopainen et al., 2014; Milliken, 2018; Sayers & de Vries, 2008). Professional touch is often about balancing beneficial and non-harmful effects and considering how optimally to do good and avoid harm to the client. Assessing the consequences of touch helps professionals to sensibly adjust their ways of touching on each occasion. The client's vulnerability is a fundamental issue that the client work professional must consider when touching, which makes professional touch a unique way of communicating with another person. A touch can have tremendous power and therefore demands a heightened sense of responsibility.

The second dimension of professionalism—touch as professional know-how—is closely related to each profession's specific, internationally shared knowledge, traditional practices, specific characteristics, objectives and normative guidelines. There is one fundamental feature: touch always starts from the client's need. For example, masseurs all over the world share the basic professional knowledge of tactile techniques and how to use therapeutic treatments with different clients. In general, professional massage therapists promise to relieve their clients' problematic symptoms and promote their overall psychophysical well-being and healthy lifestyle by responsibly applying their know-how on tactile techniques and advising the clients. Their practice is regulated by certain standards and legal guidelines in most countries, although the specific techniques require their own education and training in practice. Teachers' knowledge of touch in their work, by contrast, is intended to support children and young people's development as humans and responsible members of society, as well as providing knowledge-centred education.

All working practices, including professional touch, should be committed to these goals. Depending on the student's age, the functions and intentions of touch (Sect. 2.1) can range from a formal handshake to a hug or embrace. Early childhood educators and day care workers strive to create conditions for children to grow holistically: as part of this, physical touching guides and supports children's daily activities and provides them with feelings of safety and love.

Professional know-how on touch has become extremely important in technologised work environments, where interactions between a professional and a client increasingly involve the use of different devices or instruments, as we discuss in Chap. 4. In hospitals, for instance, touch between the nurse and the patient is frequently mediated through digital devices or research tools. We are concerned that a client's dignity and sovereignty are easily ignored in instrumental and technology-driven contact. A superficial understanding of the role of touch and technology can lead to the treatment of clients as objects. However, this need not be the case, because the nurse can apply their know-how on professional touch to making contact with the equipment feel as pleasant for the patient as possible. Consciousness of the variety of functions, possibilities, limitations and sociocultural components of touch form the core of this precious know-how. We believe that touch combined with client-driven technology guarantees the best quality of client work in the future. Body-to-body and technology-mediated practices should ideally be developed as complementary rather than contradictory working methods. The technology already in use, and the spatial and temporal resources it implies, nevertheless affect how the professional encounters a client. We argue that this is one reason for serious consideration of developing touch as a key form of professional know-how.

In touch-intensive work such as nursing, touching the patient is an everyday routine for an experienced professional in a familiar environment. But for the patient, touch is often a particular event in a strange environment, and even an apparently neutral touch from the worker may render several shades of meaning and unexpected intensities. Although the psychophysical effects of touch are at a general level well known, it is impossible to predict how different clients will respond to touch, or the ways in which they would prefer to be touched. There is an urgent need to deepen this know-how of touch, as we have noted. The secondary school teachers, wellness experts, professionals, teachers and students of healthcare and social work, whom we met repeatedly in work contexts and interviewed, often stated that different aspects of touch should be taught to students and should be an ongoing topic of education. 'Seija', a physiotherapy teacher emphasised in our interview that she has found it extremely important to teach her students about the various aspects of touch: it should be used in not only instrumental but also expressive ways.

> I teach my students that, through my presence, I hold an old [bedridden] person by the shoulder and stroke their upper arm a bit. This means a lot more to that person than talking about or telling her something. For them, words no longer matter. (Seija, Finnish physiotherapy teacher)

As we have noted previously, this opinion is no longer rare among healthcare educators. Amid the multilevel politicisation of touch and COVID-19, many professionals have struggled with the dilemmas of what kind of touch is ethically appropriate in their client interactions. The culture of client work has also changed due to digitalisation, demands for economic efficiency and the reduction of resources. But as Martina Ann Kelly and colleagues (2017) conclude from their meta-ethnography of studies across healthcare professions, touch has been the focus of surprisingly little healthcare research. Kelly and colleagues' meta-analysis focused on nurses, doctors, physiotherapists and psychotherapists, but the shortage of research is even more marked in other occupations, since nursing is the professional context where touch has been studied most.

At the same time, the topic of professional touch sometimes provokes a strange mixture of disbelief, rejection, fear, suspicion and amusement. We believe this is a result of recent scandals about abuse and harassment, as well as the oversexualisation and legal regulation of touch, which have made the topic something of a taboo. We have noticed this in some situations while giving lectures or training in professional touch. On one occasion, when we were lecturing to a group of healthcare administrative chiefs about the many potentials of touch in elderly care, one participant commented that as not all clients enjoy being touched, professionals should avoid it generally. Another stated that because touch is such an obvious means of care work, it does not need to be explicitly taught. A lecture we recently gave to professionals in forensic psychiatry was interesting in this regard. Approximately half the participants were curious to learn more about the role of touch in their clients' life courses and were open to considering its potential for their work; the other half were clearly very critical of these ideas. Sometimes, professionals agree that touch should be used more creatively and boldly in client work, but they claim it cannot be taught: either you have the natural ability to touch or you do not.

All these aspects are important. First, individual clients and workers alike have different experiences and expectations of touch, and it is important to be conscious of the differences as well as the similarities between individuals. How individuals are socialised into touch, and the learnt cultural meanings attached to touch, are in some sense involved, perhaps unconsciously, in direct tactile encounters between professionals and clients. As previously stated, body work and its institutional practices are in many ways organised by sociocultural factors. It is through primary and secondary socialisation that we get to know whom we can touch, how, when and where, and the outcomes of these socialisation processes manifest themselves as particular touching styles. Tactile life histories also resonate in the ways in which touch is psychophysically experienced and interpreted. An awareness of the sociocultural aspects of touch helps professionals to better understand their own and their clients' behaviours, attitudes, expectations and feelings related to touch, and thus to work in culturally sensitive ways. The sociocultural perspective on touch is therefore the theme of the whole of Chap. 3.

At individual and organisational levels, professionals need to be constantly developing their sensitivity skills and their awareness of different factors when they encounter clients by touching them. In addition to general professional guidelines, every organisation, whether public institution or private company, has its own distinctive working culture. Workers consciously or unconsciously absorb certain ways of touching clients, and in this way they represent and transmit their organisation's values and norms, even though an individual worker's private values may sometimes conflict with their employer's values. Touch really is such a self-evident part of so many client work tasks that we seldom think about it as a specific skill. Furthermore, it is based on intuitive and intimate bodily knowledge that is often difficult to verbalise; it is tacit knowledge, and therefore difficult to teach verbally (Parviainen, 2002). However, we believe that touch can be verbally taught and learned, based on scientific research into the functions and effects of touch and organising versatile practice.

At present, an employee's professional know-how about touch is not reflected in their salary. Indeed, researchers have observed that the more their work requires physical engagement with the client, the less pay and appreciation the employee receives. For example, in the healthcare sector, day care workers and practical nurses receive relatively low salaries. By contrast, doctors, nursing supervisors and specialist nurses, who have less physical contact with their clients, are appreciated and rewarded with higher salaries. Highly educated specialists typically communicate with clients at a distance, using written forms, digital devices or uniforms. High-status professionals focus more on client information than on direct client encounters. According to our understanding of affective work, however, knowledge about touching is not only important at the human level; it is also worthy of careful economic consideration. Touching is a skill that requires a high level of expertise and professionalism. Professional touch involves reasoning and decision-making based on embodied skills, practical wisdom and intuition. A human being is an indivisible whole made up of mind, body, knowledge and affective sensitivity, all of which are needed in professional touch.

Touch is a crucial professional skill in client work. Its adoption can no longer be left to the haphazard activity of individual workers. There is a need for a serious discussion about promoting and teaching the fruitful use of touch at work, and how to reward professionals for this professional know-how in financially fair and encouraging ways. This book will also help the professional to become more conscious of their own feelings and the affects that touch evokes in different situations and encounters. This will lead to better control and regulation of the psychophysical responses evoked by and in touch, and thus strengthen the ability to utilise touch in diverse and emotionally rewarding ways in working practices.

1.6 How to Read This Book

The content of the book is organised as follows. In Chap. 2, drawing on previous empirical and theoretical research on touch in client work, we map out seven pivotal forms of touching as embodied skill. Using examples from service industries, especially education and healthcare, we identify the following dimensions of professional touch: (1) connecting touch, (2) procedural touch, (3) assisting and guiding touch, (4) exploratory touch, (5) caring and comforting touch, (6) therapeutic touch and (7) protective and controlling touch. We show how these distinctions between the different functions of touch are justified by our aim to appreciate the full repertoire of meanings of professional touch, and that it provides a ground from which to understand and value touch's multilayered nature. At the end of the chapter, we discuss styles of professional touch that differ in their qualitative properties and capabilities, and which therefore also fulfil the multiple functions of professional touch in different ways. We emphasise the importance of 'tuning into the client's style of the flesh' when one is touching them.

Tactile encounters in client work cannot be understood or even performed unless one considers the cultural factors that are always present in encounters. Chapter 3 introduces the concept of 'skinscapes', which captures touch practices as they have developed in specific historical, ideological, economic, material and social conditions. We concentrate on primary socialisation during early childhood, and secondary socialisation with regard to how touch habits are transferred across families and generations through childcare practices. These practices produce different primary attachment styles and affective repertoires, which in turn reproduce certain touch patterns in later life. Learned affective repertoires also impact on the ways in which people encounter one another through touch in their roles as clients and professionals.

In addition to learned affective repertoires, technological devices and digital environments are pivotal to how people encounter one another through touch in their respective roles. The COVID-19 pandemic, and the digital leap that followed from it, revolutionised the touch cultures of various professions, generating touch deprivation issues. Chapter 4 focuses on technology-mediated touch in interactive client work. Drawing on critical technology studies and the phenomenology of the body, we develop a novel approach to how technological tools and digitalisation shape tactile interactions between professionals and clients. The concept of triadic touch captures the idea that technologies, tools and material objects create unpredictable affects and tensions in interactions between professionals and clients, which professionals must learn to manage.

Chapter 5 is motivated by the question: what kind of touch is ethically appropriate in an interaction with a client? We introduce novel principles of professional ethics for touch-based client work by drawing on the philosophy of ethics and research on touch and affects. This ethics considers the client's needs, but above all it rests on universal human rights, legal guidelines and professional well-being. By formulating the notion of embodied ethics, we discuss how professionals can be present to, approach or behave towards clients in fair and ethically sustainable ways, while taking account of the many factors that can limit touch interactions. In the framework of embodied ethics, the essence of touching is that one person can never touch another without being touched themselves. This reciprocity of touch has effects on professionals' work with clients, sometimes in unpredictable ways, including causing moral stress to professionals.

Chapter 6 concludes the book by looking to the future and formulating guidelines for a pedagogy that might contribute to the development of a positive touch culture in professional work. We consider different scenarios of touch cultures, and we end by discussing the central role of education in the development of professionals' touch skills.

Each chapter begins with a set of learning objectives for the topics covered. In addition, scattered throughout the chapters' main texts you will find summaries of some key themes (in boxes), key concepts (in tables) and examples (in case studies). Each chapter ends with suggested learning activities, which mainly invite you to reflect on your own experiences of touch in light of what you have read. The activities will usually take no more than 30 minutes to complete, with the exception of the fieldwork activities. The aim of the latter is to encourage you to explore more deeply the possibilities and meanings of touch in your work practices and everyday life.

There are many different ways in which you might use this book. Here are some suggestions:

- Read the whole book through (over several days) for your personal or professional use, with or without conducting the reflection activities.
- Read a specific chapter that is useful to you and only return later to the other chapters, completing the activities after each chapter if you wish.
- Use the book as core reading for a single course, or as part of one or more courses.

Above all, the book is intended for all of us who touch and are touched by the other living and non-living beings around us every day. The purpose of the book is to encourage you to deepen your understanding of touch and its hidden but multiple affective meanings, both in professional practice and in everyday life. Putting different forms of touch and related experiences into words, and discussing them with others, can often help us to identify the tacit meanings of tactile interactions.

References

Anedda, J., Ferreli, C., Rongioletti, R., & Atzori, L. (2020). Changing gears: Medical gloves in the era of coronavirus disease 2019 pandemic. *Clinics in Dermatology, 38*(6), 734–736.

Batty, C. (2015). The first sense: A philosophical study of the sense of touch. *Philosophical Psychology, 29*(1), 138–146. https://doi.org/10.1080/09515089.2015.1010197

Benner, P. (2004). Relational ethics of comfort, touch, and solace: Endangered arts? *American Journal of Critical Care, 13*(4), 346–349.

Bottorff, J. L. (1993). The use and meaning of touch in caring for patients with cancer. *Oncology Nursing Forum, 20*(10), 1531–1538.

Bush, E. (2001). The use of human touch to improve the well-being of older adults: A holistic nursing intervention. *Journal of Holistic Nursing, 19*(3), 256–270.

Cascio, C. J., Mooreb, D., & McGloneb, F. (2019). Social touch and human development. *Developmental Cognitive Neuroscience, 35*, 5–11.

Chang, E. S., & Levy, B. R. (2021). High prevalence of elder abuse during the COVID-19 pandemic: Risk and resilience factors. *The American Journal of Geriatric Psychiatry, 29*, 1152–1159. https://doi.org/10.1016/j.jagp.2021.01.007

References

Classen, C. (1993). *Worlds of sense: Exploring the senses in the history and across cultures.* Routledge.

Connor, A., & Howett, M. A. (2009). Conceptual model of intentional comfort touch. *Journal of Holistic Nursing, 27*(2), 127–135.

Cranny-Francis, A. (2011). Semefulness: A social semiotics of touch. *Social Semiotics, 21*(4), 463–481.

Davin, L., Thistlethwaite, J., Bartle, E., & Russell, K. (2019). Touch in health professional practice: A review. *The Clinical Teacher, 16*(6), 559–564. https://doi.org/10.1111/tct.13089

Dawson, A., & Dennis, S. (2021). Workplace intimacy. *Anthropology in Action, 28*(1), 1–7.

Draper, J. (2015). Embodied practice: Rediscovering the 'heart' of nursing. *Journal of Advanced Nursing, 70*(10), 2235–2244.

Driessen, A., Borgstrom, E., & Cohn, S. (2021). Ways of 'being with' caring for dying patients at the height of the COVID-19 pandemic. *Anthropology in Action, 28*(1), 16–20. https://doi.org/10.3167/aia.2021.280103

Edward, K.-L., Ousey, K., Warelow, P., & Lui, S. (2014). Nursing and aggression in the workplace: A systematic review. *British Journal of Nursing, 23*(12), 653–659.

Field, T. (Ed.). (1995). *Touch in early development.* Psychology Press.

Field, T. (2003). *Touch.* MIT Press.

Fredriksson, L. (1999). Modes of relating in a caring conversation: A research synthesis on presence, touch and listening. *Journal of Advanced Nursing, 30*(5), 1167–1176.

Fulkerson, M. (2020). Touch. In E. N. Zalta (Ed.), *The Stanford encyclopedia of philosophy* (Summer 2020 ed.). URL: https://plato.stanford.edu/archives/sum2020/entries/touch/

Fuller, B., Simmering, M. J., Marler, L. E., Cox, S. S., Bennett, R. J., & Cheramie, R. A. (2011). Exploring touch as a positive workplace behavior. *Human Relations, 64*(2), 231–256.

Gallace, A., & Spence, C. (2010). The science of interpersonal touch: An overview. *Neuroscience and Biobehavioral Reviews, 34*(2), 246–259.

García-Santesmases, A., López Gómez, D., & Pié Balaguer, A. (2022). Being just their hands? Personal assistance for disabled people as bodywork. *Sociology of Health & Illness*, 1–20. https://doi-org.pc124152.oulu.fi:9443/10.1111/1467-9566.13567

Gimlin, D. (2007). What is 'body work'? A review of the literature. *Sociology Compass, 1*(1), 353–370. https://doi.org/10.1111/j.1751-9020.2007.00015.x

Gleeson, M., & Higgins, A. (2009). Touch in mental health nursing: An exploratory study of nurses' views and perceptions. *Journal of Psychiatric and Mental Health Nursing, 16*(4), 382–389.

Green, L., & Moran, L. (2021). Covid-19, social distancing and the 'scientisation' of touch: Exploring the changing social and emotional contexts of touch and their implications for social work. *Qualitative Social Work, 20*(1–2), 171–178. https://doi.org/10.1177/1473325020973321

Gross, M. (2019). Are we losing touch with our world? *Current Biology, 29*, R265–R279.

Haho, A. (2017). Palliatiivisen vaiheen syöpäpotilaiden eksistentiaalinen kärsimys [existential suffering of cancer patients in palliative care]. *Lääkärilehti, 72*(33), 1704–1714. https://www.laakarilehti.fi/tieteessa/alkuperaistutkimukset/palliatiivisen-vaiheen-syopapotilaiden-eksistentiaalinen-karsimys/

Haho, A. (2020). *Mitä kärsimys opettaa elämästä?* [What suffering teaches about life?]. Tuuma.

Hassard, J., Holliday, R., & Willmott, H. (Eds.). (2000). *Body and organization.* Sage.

Hochschild, A. (1983). *The managed heart.* University of California Press.

Hogan, A., Thompson, G., Sellar, S., & Lingard, B. (2018). Teachers' and school leaders' perceptions of commercialisation in Australian public schools. *Australian Educational Researcher, 45*, 141–160. https://doi.org/10.1007/s13384-017-0246-7

Holopainen, G., Kasen, A., & Nyström, L. (2014). The space of togetherness – A caring encounter. *Scandinavian Journal of Caring Sciences, 28*(1), 186–192.

Howes, D. (2010). *Sensual relations: Engaging the senses in culture and social theory.* University of Michigan Press.

Hutmacher, F. (2019). Why is there so much more research on vision than on any other sensory modality? *Frontiers in Psychology, 10*, 2246. https://doi.org/10.3389/fpsyg.2019.02246

International Association of Chiefs of Police Council. (2023). https://www.theiacp.org/resources/law-enforcement-code-of-ethics

International Council of Nurses. (2021). *The ICN code of ethics for nurses.* https://www.icn.ch/system/files/2021-10/ICN_Code-of-Ethics_EN_Web_0.pdf

Irigaray, L. (1984). *Éthique de la différence sexuelle.* Éditions de Minuit.

Jablonski, N. G. (2006). *Skin: A natural history.* University of California Press.

Jakubiak, B. K., & Feeney, B. C. (2017). Affectionate touch to promote relational, psychological, and physical well-being in adulthood: A theoretical model and review of the research. *Personality and Social Psychology Review, 21*(3), 228–252.

Johansen, T. K. (1997). *Aristotle on the sense-organs.* Cambridge University Press.

Jütte, R. (2005). *The history of the senses. From antiquity to cyberspace.* Polity Press.

Kahsay, W. G., Negarandeh, R., Nayeri, N. D., & Hasanpour, M. (2020). Sexual harassment against female nurses: A systematic review. *BMC Nursing, 19*(58). https://doi.org/10.1186/s12912-020-00450-w

Kelly, M. A., Nixon, L., McClurg, C., Scherpbier, A., King, N., & Dornan, T. (2017). Experience of touch in healthcare: A meta-ethnography across the healthcare professions. *Qualitative Health Research,* 1–13. https://doi.org/10.1177/1049732317707726

Keltner, D. (2009). *Born to be good. The science of a meaningful life.* .

Kinnunen, T. (2013). *Vahvat yksin, heikot sylityksin. Otteita suomalaisesta kosketuskulttuurista* [Strong ones alone, weak ones in each others' laps]. Kirjapaja.

Kinnunen, T., & Kolehmainen, M. (2019). Touch and affect. Analysing the archive of touch biographies. *Body & Society, 25*(1), 29–56.

Kinnunen, T., & Parviainen, J. (2016). Feeling the right personality. Recruitment Consultants' affective decision making in interviews with employee candidates. *Nordic Journal of Working Life Studies, 6*(3), 5–21.

Kinnunen, T., & Seppänen, J. (2009). Oikeaoppinen opettajaruumis. *Naistutkimus, 4,* 6–17.

Kinnunen, T., Parviainen, J., Haho, A., & Jolkkonen, M. (2019). *Ammatillinen kosketus. Kuinka tunnetyötä tehdään* [Professional touch. Affective work in practice]. Kirjapaja.

Lafrance, M. (2018). Skin studies: Past, present and future. *Body & Society, 24*(1–2), 3–32.

Lanoix, M. (2013). Labor as embodied practice: The lessons of care work. *Hypatia, 28*(1), 85–100.

Lanoix, M. (2019). Un amour de robot: Robot émotionnel et travail d'aidant. In M.-H. Parizeau & S. Kash (Eds.), *La société robotisée. Enjeux éthiques et politiques* (pp. 259–279). Presses de l'Université Laval.

Löken, L., Wessberg, J., Morrison, I., McGlone, F., & Olaussonet, H. (2009). Coding of pleasant touch by unmyelinated afferents in humans. *Nature Neuroscience, 12*(5), 547–548. https://doi.org/10.1038/nn.2312

Lopez, S. H. (2006). Culture change management in long-term care: A shop-floor view. *Politics and Society, 34*(1), 55–80. https://doi.org/10.1177/0032329205284756

Manning, E. (2007). *Politics of touch: Sense, movement, sovereignty.* University of Minnesota Press.

Milliken, A. (2018). Ethical awareness: What it is and why it matters? *The Online Journal of Issues in Nursing, 23*(1). https://doi.org/10.3912/OJIN.Vol23No01Man01

Montagu, A. (1971). *Touching.* Columbia University Press.

Nätynki, P., Kinnunen, T., & Kolehmainen, M. (2023). Embracing water, healing pine: Touch-walking and transcorporeal worldings. *Senses & Society.* https://doi.org/10.1080/17458927.2180864

Nazarko, L. (2020). COVID-19 and gloves: When to wear and when not to wear. *British Journal of Healthcare Assistants, 14*(4), 185–189.

Nist, M. D., Harrison, T. M., Tate, J., Robinson, A., Balas, M., & Pickler, R. H. (2020). Losing touch. *Nursing Inquiry, 27,* e12368.

Obrador, P. (2012). Touching the beach. In M. Paterson & M. Dodge (Eds.), *Touching space, placing touch* (pp. 47–70). Routledge.

Parviainen, J. (2002). Bodily knowledge: Epistemological reflections on dance. *Dance Research Journal, 34*(1), 11–23. https://doi.org/10.2307/1478130

Parviainen, J. (2014). The performativity of "double bodies": Exploring the phenomenological conception of *Leib/Körper* distinction in interactive bodywork. *The International Journal of Work Organisation and Emotion, 6*(4), 311–326. https://doi.org/10.1504/IJWOE.2014.068031

Parviainen, J. (2018). Embodying industrial knowledge: An epistemological approach to the formation of body knowledge in the context of the fitness industry. *The Sociology of Sport Journal, 35*(4), 358–366. https://doi.org/10.1123/ssj.2017-0168

Parviainen, J., & Aromaa, J. (2017). Bodily knowledge beyond motor skills and physical fitness: A phenomenological description of knowledge formation in physical training. *Sport, Education and Society, 22*(4), 477–492. https://doi.org/10.1080/13573322.2015.1054273

Parviainen, J., & Kortelainen, I. (2019). Becoming fully present in your body: Analysing mindfulness as an affective investment in tech culture. *Somatechnics, 9*(2–3), 353–375. https://doi.org/10.3366/soma.2019.0288

Parviainen, J., & Pirhonen, J. (2017). Vulnerable bodies in human-robot interaction: Embodiment as ethical issue in robot care for the elderly. *Transformation, 29*, 104–115.

Parviainen, J., Turja, T., & Van Aerschot, L. (2019). Social robots and human touch in care: The perceived usefulness of robot assistance among healthcare professionals. In O. Korn (Ed.), *Social robots. An interdisciplinary compendium on technological, societal and ethical aspects* (pp. 533–540). Springer.

Paterson, M. (2007). *The senses of touch: Haptics, affects and technologies*. Bloomsbury.

Puroila, A.-M., & Haho, A. (2017). Moral functioning: Navigating the messy landscape of values in Finnish preschools. *Scandinavian Journal of Educational Research, 61*(5), 540–554. https://doi.org/10.1080/00313831.2016.1172499

Rajan-Rankin, S. (2018). Invisible bodies and disembodied voices? Identity work, the body and embodiment in transnational service work. *Gender, Work and Organization, 25*(1), 9–23.

Ratcliffe, M. (2012). What is touch? *Australasian Journal of Philosophy, 90*(3), 413–432. https://doi.org/10.1080/00048402.2011.598173

Roberts, T. (2020). COVID-19 and touch deprivation. *PsychCentral, 29*. https://psychcentral.com/blog/covid-19-and-touch-deprivation/

Saarinen, A., Harjunen, V., Jasinskaja-Lahti, I., Jääskeläinen, I. P., & Ravaja, N. (2021). Social touch experience in different contexts: A review. *Neuroscience and Biobehavioral Reviews, 131*, 360–372.

Sayers, K. L., & de Vries, K. (2008). A concept development of 'being sensitive' in nursing. *Nursing Ethics, 15*(3), 289–303.

Schellekens, E. (2009). Taste and objectivity: The emergence of the concept of the aesthetic. *Philosophy Compass, 4*, 734–743. https://doi.org/10.1111/j.1747-9991.2009.00234.x

Skountridaki, L. (2019). The patient–doctor relationship in the transnational healthcare context. *Sociology of Health & Illness, 41*(8), 1685–1705.

Sunanta, S. (2020). Globalising the Thai 'high-touch' industry: Exports of care and body work and gendered mobilities to and from Thailand. *Journal of Ethnic and Migration Studies, 46*(4), 1–19. https://doi.org/10.1080/1369183X.2020.1711568

Twigg, J. (2006). *The body in health and social care*. Palgrave Macmillan.

Twigg, J., Wolkowitz, C., Cohen, R. L., & Nettleton, S. (2011). Conceptualising body work in health and social care. *Sociology of Health & Illness, 33*(2), 171–188. https://doi.org/10.1111/j.1467-9566.2010.01323.x. Epub 2011 Jan 12. PMID: 21226736.

Uno, M. (2021). Patient-nurse conflict: Verification of structural model. In S. Durmus (Ed.), *Nursing: New perspectives* (pp. 63–84). IntecOpen.

Uvnäs Moberg, K. (2003). *The oxytocin factor: Tapping the hormone of calm, love, and healing*. Da Capo Press.

Vallbo, Å., Olausson, H., Wessberg, J., & Norrsell, U. (1993). A system of unmyelinated afferents for innocuous mechanoreception in the human skin. *Brain Research, 628*(1–2), 301–304. https://doi.org/10.1016/0006-8993(93)90968-S. PMID 8313159. S2CID 29606427.

Van Aerschot, L., & Parviainen, J. (2020). Robots responding to care needs? A multitasking care robot pursued for 25 years, available products offer simple entertainment and instrumental assistance. *Ethics and Information Technology, 22*, 247–256. https://doi.org/10.1007/s10676-020-09536-0

Van Dongen, E., & Elema, R. (2001). The art of touching: The culture of 'body work' in nursing. *Anthropology & Medicine, 8*(2–3), 149–162.

Van Keer, R. L., Deschepper, R., Francke, A. L., Huyghens, L., & Bilsen, J. (2015). Conflicts between healthcare professionals and families of a multi-ethnic patient population during critical care: An ethnographic study. *Critical Care, 19*, 441. https://doi.org/10.1186/s13054-015-1158-4

Weeks, K. (2007). Life within and against work: Affective labor, feminist critique, and post-Fordist politics. *Ephemera: Theory and Politics in Organization, 7*(1), 233–249.

WHO. (2022). *A guide to WHO's guidance on COVID-19*. https://www.who.int/news-room/feature-stories/detail/a-guide-to-who-s-guidance

Wilk, S., Siegl, L., Siegl, K., & Hohenstein, C. (2018). Miscommunication as a risk focus in patient safety: Work process analysis in prehospital emergency care. *Der Anaesthesist, 67*(4), 255–263. https://doi.org/10.1007/s00101-018-0413-x. PMID: 29404658.

Witz, A., Warhurst, C., & Nickson, D. (2003). The labour of aesthetics and the aesthetics of organization. *Organization, 10*(1), 33–54.

Wolf, Z. R., Bailey, D. N., & Stubin, C. A. (2022). Bodywork and nursing practice: Development of a bodywork in nursing practice instrument. *Nursing Forum, 57*, 509–529. https://doi.org/10.1111/nuf.12703

Wolkowitz, C. (2006). *Bodies at work*. Sage Publications.

Yon, Y., Mikton, C. R., Gassoumis, Z. D., & Wilber, K. H. (2017). Elder abuse prevalence in community settings: A systematic review and meta-analysis. *The Lancet Global Health, 5*, e147–e156. https://doi.org/10.1016/S2214-109X(17)30006-2

Touch as a Professional Skill

2

Abstract

This chapter introduces (1) connecting touch, (2) procedural touch, (3) assisting and guiding touch, (4) exploratory touch, (5) caring and comforting touch, (6) therapeutic touch and (7) protective and controlling touch. The classification is necessary to encompass the whole repertoire of professional touch, although the chapter demonstrates how the various functions merge and change during typical work routines. We frame this discussion with theoretical outlines regarding the body's relationality in touch. The varying meanings of touch stem from its heightened situational nature and its status as part of wider multisensory communication. This chapter considers techniques and styles of professional touch that differ in their qualitative properties and capabilities. We analyse what these qualitative distinctions are from the perspectives of clients and professionals themselves. The last section focuses on the importance of tuning into the client's 'style of the flesh' when one is touching them.

Introduction

This chapter considers touch as a part of 'soft skills' by first introducing the different functions of professional touch. We distinguish (1) connecting touch, (2) procedural touch, (3) assisting and guiding touch, (4) exploratory touch, (5) caring and comforting touch, (6) therapeutic touch, and (7) protective and controlling touch. This classification is our own, but it is largely inspired by earlier research, especially research conducted by nursing scientists, who have been creating taxonomies of touch in care work for decades. We also utilise other previous empirical and theoretical research on touch in client work, body work and human communication to map out the multiple skills, roles and outcomes that touch can have in working practices, without clients or professionals being fully conscious of them.

We argue that our classification is necessary to encompass the whole repertoire of professional touch. Discussing the different functions of touch also provides us with a basis from which to understand touch's multilayered nature and its value as a professional soft skill. However, we emphasise that any strict separation between the different functions of touch will always be somewhat artificial and arbitrary. Using examples from our own research materials, as well as other research findings and illustrations from everyday life, we demonstrate how touch's various functions and intentions merge and change during typical work routines. We frame this discussion with theoretical outlines regarding the body's relationality in touch—the body's fluid boundaries, and its ambiguous position as both affecting another body and being affected by it. We stress that the varying meanings of touch stem from its heightened situational nature and its status as part of wider multisensory communication.

The last sections of the chapter discuss techniques and styles of professional touch that differ in their qualitative properties and capabilities, and which therefore also fulfil the multiple functions of professional touch in different ways. We analyse what these qualitative distinctions are from the perspectives of clients and professionals themselves; we also discuss the potential consequences of these touch styles and interactions for clients. The last section focuses on the importance of tuning into the client's 'style of the flesh' when one is touching them. However, this demands a consciousness of one's own style, as well as the sensitivity required to register the impulses and affects that move across bodies in professional encounters.

Learning Objectives
With reasonable effort on your part, by the end of the chapter you will be able to:

- Identify seven different functions of professional touch in terms of the intentions or aims of the professionals who use touch as a working tool.
- Discuss styles of professional touch that differ from one another in their qualitative properties.
- Describe the kinds of work task in which touch is an essential working tool and the key channel for communication with the client.
- Explain why touch is a powerful vehicle for expressing emotions and transmitting affects across bodies.

2.1 Mapping Multidimensional Functions of Professional Touch

> Touch is not thought to be a part of professionalism. Touch should be broken down into small enough pieces to start seeing the wood for the trees. If you don't understand touch, you don't fully appreciate your own profession. After all, through touch, it pops up when you value your own profession and the way you work. This is all realised there in the well-being of our residents as well. (Rebekka, Finnish practical nurse)

Rebekka, who worked as a practical nurse in geriatric ward, gave an interesting summary of her thoughts about the importance of touch in her work. During our interview, she suggested that touch should be 'broken down into pieces' so that one could understand its multitude of crucial roles in care work. In what follows, we will do exactly that by mapping numerous ways of utilising touch in nursing and other forms of body work. Indeed, nursing scientists have been breaking touch down into pieces for decades. There are various taxonomies of touch, distinguishing for example between caring, protective and task-oriented touch (Estabrooks, 1989; Estabrooks & Morse, 1992; Papathanassoglou & Mpouzika, 2012; Routasalo, 1999). Caring touch is typically understood as comforting or encouraging, and as analogous to 'expressive' or 'affectional' touch. It is also associated with emotional spontaneity and is considered to diverge from task-oriented 'instrumental' touch (Bush, 2001; Davin et al., 2019; Gleeson & Higgins, 2009). While refined versions of such taxonomies can range from a few to well over a hundred categories of touch, they all make this rough division between *procedural* touch (also called e.g. 'necessary', 'instrumental', 'functional' or 'task-oriented') and *non-procedural* touch (also called e.g. 'non-necessary', 'expressive', 'therapeutic', 'emotional', 'affectional', 'caring', 'connecting' or 'comforting') (e.g. Bush, 2001; Chang, 2001; Gleeson & Higgins, 2009; Kelly et al., 2017; Wolf et al., 2022).

Corresponding categorisations have presumably not been made with regard to other fields of client work, although the distinction between procedural and non-procedural (or 'communicative') touch has been applied to studies of touch in medicine, physiotherapy and occupational therapy, for example (Kelly et al., 2017, p. 4). For Virve Keränen and her research partners (2017), who have studied the tactile practices of early childhood education professionals, the main distinction is between 'unconscious' and 'conscious pedagogical touch'. The latter refers to the child's multifaceted collaboration and participatory touch. The functions of touch naturally vary between professions. Nursing is largely based on the performance of necessary procedures, whereas in social work, policing and security guard work, touch is often an impulsive and coercive means of protection for the client, the professional or others. It is also notable that in much of the work in the social, educational, artistic and sports fields, as well as in some types of healthcare, tactile contact with clients is discretionary. This does not apply to most of the professionals discussed in this book, for whom touch is an essential working tool. For dentists or other procedure-focused medical specialists (e.g. ophthalmic or ear, nose and throat specialists), and for nurses who work in laboratories or the emergency services, it is impossible to carry out their work tasks without touch mediated by an instrument or technology.

Researchers into professional touch have pointed out that touch bears nuanced meanings that are always interpreted *in context*. Luke Tanner (2017), who has studied the use of touch in dementia care, lists four factors that are fundamental to the experience of touch: (1) the type of touch (e.g. the quality and duration of touch, the part of the body being touched); (2) the situation of touch (why, where and when the touch occurs, the intention and circumstances of the touch); (3) the tactile relationship (attributes of the individuals involved in the touch); (4) body language (proximity and multisensory communication). Besides the factors Tanner mentions, other studies have proposed that, e.g. individual personality styles, the reciprocity of touch, cultural variables, the seriousness of the situation, and the presence of contagious conditions can influence patterns, interpretations and experiences of touch in client work encounters (Bush, 2001; Dawson & Dennis, 2021; Estabrooks, 1989; O'Lynn & Krautscheid, 2011). Not only do experiences and interpretations of touch vary significantly between clients, but their expectations, hopes and doubts about a professional's manner of touching can also be diverse.

So, whose perspective should be the starting point to determine even the most basic distinction between 'necessary' and 'unnecessary' touch? Might the assertion of such a dichotomy even be harmful (Douglas, 2021)? It is clear that we lack exact criteria for different functions of professional touch, and we will consider several aspects of the complex contextual meanings of touch in later chapters. However, we stress that rough distinctions provide a comprehensive picture of the multiple functions of touch in client work and serve as a useful analytical tool to discuss them. They highlight the multitude of different *work tasks* and the professionals' related *intentions* of touching. Further, distinctions help us to grasp the multiple *meanings* and *experiences* of touch in client encounters, which may be individual or shared by the professional and their client, and may be vibrant, volatile and sometimes ambiguous in nature.

The Finnish practical nurse Rebekka also thought that talking explicitly about touch would increase the general awareness and appreciation of care work, which in turn would naturally boost nurses' professional pride and in doing so would also benefit clients. We agree. In the era of the service economy and its increased 'emotionalisation' and 'aestheticisation' of (body) labour (see Gimlin, 2007), client work experts are expected to manage their embodied presentations and emotional performances—including their touch skills—for the purpose of pleasing the client. The ability to touch clients properly in different situations for different purposes while following professional feeling rules (see Sect. 1.3) is one of the soft skills implicitly demanded of female client workers in particular, often with no acknowledgement of how demanding this actually is (Cain, 2017). Indeed, teachers, social workers and healthcare professionals find themselves at the meeting point of a wide range of requirements. They are expected to carry out an ever-increasing number of mandatory tasks, often with decreasing resources, and also to offer 'human extras' to shore up the competitiveness of the organisation they represent. Professionalism with regard to touch should permeate every dimension of professional competence, even though it is not always fully recognised. We therefore think that distinguishing different functions of touch enables us to grasp the whole spectrum of competences held by professionals who use touch as their working tool.

In sum, 'breaking touch down into pieces' helps us to understand touch's vital multiple roles in client work—to grasp its full functional repertoire, and thus hopefully to further value it as an embodied working skill. In the following discussion, we combine previous research with our own reflections.

2.1.1 Connecting Touch

Touch in the form of greeting behaviour is an important human (and non-human) way to open oneself to communication and create mutual trust (Box 2.1). Shaking hands, or touching one another's hands in some other way, is the most typical greeting gesture in many cultures, especially when people are meeting for the first time. It marks the beginning and end of an encounter (Klopf & McCroskey, 2007, p. 229), but it can also be used as 'tactile tactic' (Box 2.2). Of course, there are

> **Box 2.1 Rapid Touch in Customer Service**
> Touch can be a powerful way to influence others' decision-making and give an impression of sincerity. Observational studies based on empirical experiments have demonstrated that a light and rapid (one- or two-second) touch during a fleeting encounter is an effective way to influence a stranger's behaviour. People are more willing to spare some change for a street person, leave a tip in a restaurant, return a book to a library, sign a petition or fill in a complicated questionnaire if they are touched on the arm or shoulder by the requester or service provider. In the same way, touch increases compliance with commercial or courtship requests and encourages people to help others in various situations (Camps et al., 2013; Fuller et al., 2011; Guèguen, 2007). However, the effects of a stranger's touch must not be understood as unidirectional manipulation. Rather, a pleasant touch, even from a stranger, can promote well-being, encourage pro-relational dyadic behaviours such as helping and cooperation, and synergistically benefit both sides in the encounter (see Jakubiak & Feeney, 2017, pp. 7–8).

> **Box 2.2 Tactile Tactics in Business**
> As anthropologist Sarah Hillewaert (2016, p. 24) suggests, a handshake can be a 'tactile tactic', 'a tool that is embodied and culturally scripted as well as consciously manipulated'. In public performances, a handshake is often meant to signal friendship, trust, equality and a willingness to collaborate. However, sometimes it can resemble a public power struggle between two powerful persons. Former US president Donald Trump became famous for his special handshake grip. With a 'jerk and pull' movement, he would stretch out his hand for a handshake but then suddenly pull his partner's hand towards him, often with the result that the partner had to bend or lean forwards as if making a bow. While he was president, Trump's handshakes with other heads of state would last for an exaggeratedly long time. We especially remember his encounters with French president Emmanuel Macron: their hands would grip so hard their knuckles would turn white, and their jaws clenched. Macron, however, is generally known for his heartily performed greetings—kissing, hugging or putting his arms around the other person, be they a president or a prime minister.

remarkable cultural and work-related variations in how greeting touches can happen. Although we can posit (with slight reservations) that some gestures and touchable body areas are cross-cultural (Suvilehto et al., 2019), there are cultural differences regarding, for example, whether one is expected to hold or shake hands, kiss one another on the cheek, beard or forehead, or refrain from any touch at all (e.g. Field, 2003, pp. 21–22). Therefore, cultural differences must be considered during all phases of the client encounter, from the greeting to the farewell (see Sect. 3.2). 'Pekka', a Finnish nurse who had worked in Saudi Arabia, gave an illuminating example of learning to conduct forms of greeting in his professional role that differed from his own learned style. He wrote about his experience in his touch biography:

I shook hands with the patients' male family members as much as five times a day. They could come within thirty centimetres of me, touch my shoulder or chest. You soon get used to that anyway – you must respect their way. A grateful patient or family member could even kiss my cheek or forehead, the way they greet good friends, relatives or respected persons. As such, there was of course nothing sexual in their touch. It was only cultural etiquette. A hand on my shoulder told me that he respects me. A hand on my chest meant that he respects me both as a person and as a nurse and trusts me – and leaves his loved ones in my care. (Pekka, Finnish nurse)

A connecting touch is like a business card the professional leaves with the client: it sets the direction for the whole appointment. In healthcare contexts in particular, handshakes are sometimes avoided to minimise the risk of infection, as became well known during the COVID-19 pandemic. However, a touch of some kind, be it a handshake, a hug or a pat on the shoulder, is a fruitful way for a professional to build a connection with the client. In a study conducted in Ireland, nurses stated that when they met a client for the first time, they would shake hands with the intention of 'trying to develop some sort of rapport with them and then take it from there'. These nurses thought that touch 'breaks down a barrier between the patient and the nurse', makes the patient 'feel that you're concerned and interested in what they are saying', and 'displays some kind of humanity' (Gleeson & Higgins, 2009).

The nurses we interviewed thought that a greeting touch in the form of a handshake was a polite habit that would get an encounter off to a good start, especially if they did not already know the client beforehand. The interviewees also mentioned touching one or both shoulders, an arm or a hand as typical ways to greet a client. According to our observations, many hairdressers and beauticians also tend to hug their regular clients, both when they enter the salon and when they leave. If the encounter involves the client lying on a treatment table in a beautician's or masseur's treatment room, the professional may greet the client by touching their shoulder, foot or other body part, just to show attention and respect. In many jobs, the connection with the client is expected to be rebuilt repeatedly, perhaps many times a day. For example, a day care nurse may grab a child by the hand several times a day to recreate a safe connection, or a nurse may touch a dementia patient lightly on the shoulder each time before starting to help them with daily tasks.

As a basic rule, clients also expect professionals to greet them with a touch that makes them feel welcome, accepted, noticed, respected and secure. Severely ill patients have described how the touch of a professional helps them to feel 'whole' and recognised as complete, vibrant individuals rather than 'invalids' (Leonard & Kalman, 2015). In a study conducted in the US, one patient summarised the importance of establishing rapport before the professional starts to touch any intimate body parts during a care procedure: 'Establish a relationship with the patient. Tell me your name. Tell me what's the next plan of action. Make a human connection' (O'Lynn & Krautscheid, 2011).

There are people who have been diagnosed with 'tactile defensiveness', a neurological disorder that manifests itself in withdrawal from touch, increased motor responses or aggressive behaviours (Royeen & Mu, 2003). However, there are probably extremely few clients who would derive the most benefit from not being touched at all. Rather, the main problem is that the importance of connecting touch is not fully understood in relation to some clients, such as psychiatric patients. Since psychiatric patients often conduct their own physical care, procedural touching is not necessarily a part of their daily care routines (Gleeson & Higgins, 2009). Combined with many psychiatric professionals' deliberate caution about touching their clients in general (e.g. Hunter & Struve, 1998), this means that many psychiatric patients receive no touch of any kind from professionals, even when they need it. For these reasons, we would very strongly emphasise the importance of connecting touch in work with psychiatric clients. There are situations in psychiatric care where touch can be used to replace words if the latter seem to be limited, inadequate or unnecessary, as an Irish psychiatric nurse described:

They just don't want to talk, they just want a bit of reassurance… maybe putting your hand on their shoulder, or maybe sometimes putting your hand over their hand and saying 'look I'm here, if you want to talk I'll listen'. (An Irish nurse, quoted in Gleeson & Higgins, 2009, p. 386)

2.1.2 Procedural Touch

When a person enters a hospital or a nursing home, the body becomes a terrain of medical practices and care. This implies that the body is an object external to the self and will be subjected to the authority of others: physicians and nurses. These others and also the self deal with the malfunctioning parts of the body, not with the body as such. This mechanism allows people to touch and to be touched in a way which is considered inappropriate and a matter out of place in another context. The body is experienced as something one has, not as a body one is. (Van Dongen & Elema, 2001, p. 153)

In this extract, Els Van Dongen and Riekje Elema acknowledge that the patient's body (or its parts) is treated as an object of care and medical procedures in hospital-like contexts where professionals have permission to touch bodies in ways that would be unacceptable elsewhere. It has been estimated that about 95% of tactile nursing practices are related to procedural touch. This includes procedures performed with the help of various aids and technical devices, such as measuring blood sugar or blood pressure, taking a blood sample, giving an injection, cannulating a blood vessel, inserting a urinary catheter, and applying or removing a dressing (McCann & McKenna, 1993). Further, nursing tasks in surgery, emergency care, intensive care and x-ray units, for example, include a versatile spectrum of procedural touch tasks, while the work of a practical nurse involves a remarkable amount of hygiene care.

According to our interviewees, practical touch is usually the only form of professional touch that is learned in nursing education and included on the curriculum. It is considered mainly from the perspective of technical performance and the proper way of 'intruding' into the client's personal space (cf. Dobson et al., 2002). Patients often fear certain kinds of procedures in advance, a fear they may express by making gestures of withdrawal or revulsion, sweating, trembling, engaging in nervous play or bursting into tears. They may feel dubious about the competence of the professional or the functioning of the technological aids and devices. Therefore, it is important to warn the client about all the unpleasant sensations the procedure might generate, such as the professional's cold hands, the damp feel of the gloves, or the pinch or tremble of a technical device. Further, it is necessary to describe to the client how and why the procedure is going to be performed, and then to report on each phase of the procedure. Tactful wording is important, including with memory-impaired clients, even if there is no certainty that they will understand.

Disposable gloves, together with aprons and face, eye and mouth protection, are an institutionally recommended form of safe contact between practitioners and clients in healthcare. Such protection is used to prevent the transmission of microorganisms through body fluids, secretions and excretions, or contaminated instruments. Professionals navigate creatively between institutional guidelines, personal intuition and affective relationalities, while aiming to ensure that their encounters with clients are not only physically safe but also morally sustainable (Pink et al., 2014). However, the use of gloves also carries different meanings. Professionals are often worried about the 'unjustified' use of gloves. The nurses we interviewed, for example, said they were shocked by cases they had witnessed where doctors or other nurses had used gloves with no medical justification. In their view, this was purely distancing behaviour—perhaps even 'intentional emotional coldness' or a sign of very limited emotional resources—which they perceived as unprofessional and ethically problematic.

Another ethical dilemma associated with procedural touch is how to handle one's mandatory obligations to clients while respecting their right to integrity and inviolability (Chang, 2001). With the exception of certain emergency situations, the intention behind the professional's touch should always be grounded in the client's permission insofar as the client must have the opportunity to negotiate about how they are touched by the professional, or indeed to refuse to be touched at all. Our nursing specialist interviewees spontaneously brought up the example of urinary catheterisation as an ordinary procedure that patients typically fear and often resist. The pain can be relieved by local anaesthetic as well as a soothing touch before the catheterisation. However, according to the interviewees, not all nurses always used local anaesthesia correctly, and some did not bother to calm or comfort the patient before the procedure; our interviewees considered this to be ethically intolerable negligence. Some nurses think that most procedures should only be performed at all if the client has understood and accepted it, at least to some degree. At the same time, of course, every nurse understands that certain procedures need to be performed one way or another. Nurses therefore strive to develop creative ways to make clients feel comfortable and not to violate their dignity, even in the most challenging situations.

Tasks related to the management of intimate hygiene evoked a lot of reflection in our interviews. Such management includes washing intimate body parts and changing underwear and incontinence pads. Although the tasks are routine for practical nurses working in elderly care, for example, they must repeatedly attune themselves to clients who need time to adjust to their situation, and the clients who resist such tasks at first must be treated sensitively. It is extremely difficult for some clients to accept their new situation. The hygiene procedures may feel unpleasant, embarrassing or even humiliating to the patient, and it is not uncommon for the client and the nurse to disagree about the need for a change of underwear. This entails convincing the client about the facts because, as one practical nurse put it, 'of course, you have to take care of the person and clean up, and tell them that you can't sit in the dirt'. Here again, no matter what the situation may be, one must always warn the client when one is about to undo their clothing. Some of our nurse interviewees thought it worth avoiding talking about the incontinence pads and talking instead about 'changing into dry pants'. They said that 'nappy' was a word that could evoke deep feelings of shame, especially among male clients.

The time spent performing procedures and the rhythm of the work are crucial qualitative elements of necessary touch. Hectic working conditions often mean that professionals carry out routines without paying sufficient attention or respect to the client's bodily rhythms. However, as many of our interviewees stressed, if the professional can stop for a moment and synchronise their own rhythm with that of the client, this can actually shorten the time required for the procedure. Sometimes it is better to wait until the client is ready for a necessary procedure, whether that takes ten minutes or half an hour, as our nurse interviewees stated. This attitude was also perceived as the mark of a true professional and a matter of ethical choice.

Some nurses take task-oriented touch as an opportunity to encounter the client holistically, which involves consciously thinking about how the necessary procedures are to be performed. 'Jonna', who worked as a practical nurse in home care, told us that for her, a caring and even beautifying touch would ideally be combined with the normal routines of washing the client's body and hair. She was pleased that her current job gave her the opportunity to do this, unlike her previous job on a health centre ward:

> Here I care about the clients, all from start to finish. I wash their heads and wash their bodies, and put on skin cream afterwards. I may even do their hair and give them a cuddle when I leave. On the ward, all the patient work has become such a conveyor belt. You don't have the time to be present to the person as you would want to be. It's just bop, bop, bop, pads and clothes off and on, and hair after that, and on to the next one. (Jonna, Finnish practical nurse)

Consistent with previous studies (e.g. Gleeson & Higgins, 2009; Leonard & Kalman, 2015), our nurse interviewees found it problematic when instrumental touch was used in an 'uncaring' or 'robotic' way. They thought that touch could even be detrimental if it was 'urgent', 'harsh' or 'absent' and caused an unpleasant situation for both the care recipient and the caregiver. This reminds us of some scandalous maltreatment cases and the constant lack of sufficient resources in services for older and disabled people, a problem reported in many countries (Yon et al., 2017) that was quickly exacerbated during the COVID-19 pandemic (Chang & Levy, 2021). In some care units, intimate hygiene and compulsory measures in general are barely taken care of at all. In such cases, we can speak of severe violations of human rights.

2.1.3 Assisting and Guiding Touch

Nurses, physiotherapists and occupational therapists, primary schoolteachers, personal assistants for disabled people, social workers, physical education teachers, athletics coaches and dance teachers all use assistive and guiding touch in their working routines. In work with young children, older adults, and people with sensory impairments, touch has an important role in accompanying, supporting and directing the movements of the client's body so that the client feels they are coping safely with different tasks and situations (Box 2.3). For instance, a nurse can make remarkable use of assisting touch with a client who has recently lost their sight. 'Sari', a practical nurse who worked in home care, described to us what assistive touch in daily activities with such a client entailed: guiding the client's hand with her own to show where the cutlery was on the table; putting the client's hand on the edge of the sink, and moving it in the right direction while they shaved and performed other hygiene routines.

Cooking, serving and eating meals and taking oral medication are typical tasks where many older people in particular need an assisting touch, regardless of whether they live in their own home, a care home or a hospital unit. Assistive touch is often

> **Box 2.3 Lifting Patients Using the Kinaesthetics Method**
> In all situations of assisting touch, the professional's grip should be safe and competent, both to give the client confidence and to be ergonomically safe for the professional themselves. Organisations are increasingly developing work practices that help professionals assist, move and transfer clients efficiently and appropriately. Kinaesthetic care is a nursing method that aims to prevent work-related spine disorders and to make the patient feel comfortable during the transfer situation. Etymologically, 'kinaesthesia' comes from the Greek words *kinēma* (movement) and *aisthētikōs* (perceptual, receptive, sensory). Kinaesthetics was developed in the early 1970s by Lenny Maietta and Frank White Hatch in Central Europe. Together with registered nurse Suzanne Bernard Schmidt, Maietta and Hatch developed a job-specific programme called 'Kinaesthetics in nursing'. Professionals help patients by using spiral rather than parallel movements because the former require less effort. Thus, the skilful and economical use of the body puts as little strain on the caregiver's own body as possible, while the transfer makes the patient feel safe and comfortable (Freiberg et al., 2016; Fringer et al., 2014). Being able to choose the best possible grips in different situations requires empathic awareness of one's own and others' body postures, breathing and movements. Caregivers thus need training in body awareness to cope with day-to-day assistance and care situations.

also used to help the client to move from one place to another, such as getting out of a bed or chair and going to the bathroom. With some clients, the professional must lead them by the hand; with others, it is enough to support them from behind. The client may use a technical aid for moving, such as a wheelchair, walking stick or walking frame, while the caregiver walks next to them and gently touches their back to give them a sense of security. An illness can cause temporary or permanent functional impairment for clients of all ages and give rise to the need for an assisting touch in daily tasks.

The core idea behind assisting touch is to encourage and support the client's own ability to perform the task in question. Assistive touch should thus not turn into a purely instrumental touch in the sense that the client's own activity is denied or the procedure is not sufficiently explained to the client beforehand. The accelerated pace of work often sets the professional's rhythm in such a way that there are barely any temporal resources to deal with the client holistically or engage with the core idea of assisting touch. It may be easier for the caregiver to carry out the whole task themselves than it would be to patiently assist the client to perform the task, whether in collaboration or by themselves in their own manner and rhythm.

The focus of assistive touch may be on *rehabilitation*: to improve or at least maintain the client's physical capabilities. Physiotherapists and occupational therapists are rehabilitative touch professionals with expertise in a wide range of techniques and methods that are carried out by touch. Rehabilitative touch is used to support and promote the client's ability to move, cope independently and manage their own life. However, as a person's functionality weakens and their need for help increases, so does their need for various assisting touches from caregivers. In a situation where a weakened client can no longer get out of bed, all the treatments and assisted tasks are carried out on the bed. At this stage, position management plays a central role, preventing pressure ulcers and relieving the anxiety of the assisted person. Assistive touch also plays a key role in work with a very different kind of client: small children. The younger the child, the more they are assisted, supported and guided through touch. Touch in nursery schools or other day care sites is related to putting on or removing clothes, eating, playing, or other activities. The aim is to gradually teach the child to become self-oriented and autonomous in daily routines.

Guiding touch can be regarded as a form of assistive touch where a coach, personal trainer, or dance or fitness instructor guides the client through motor movements. A fitness instructor or yoga teacher may help practitioners to perform movements so that they are effective and correctly targeted at certain body parts. In some classes, such as Pilates and yoga, the instructor may use touch to help practitioners achieve the proper poses (known in yoga as 'asanas'). In her study of the use of touch during Pilates instruction, Dominika Czarnecka (2020) found that instructors often use touch to correct practitioners' exercising. Similarly, a golf coach, for example, may use assistive touch to help the client to achieve the correct trajectory with their entire body for different shots. Sports practitioners are also typically guided to ensure that they align their moves correctly without harming their bodies. In some sports, such as yoga, teachers must have an in-depth knowledge of anatomy and personal expertise in the discipline so that they can support the student's body in the 'opening' of asanas. By 'opening', yoga practitioners mean the ability to complete a posture that one could not do previously. If the teacher does not provide help correctly, this can lead to injuries caused by a disregard of the body's signals.

Dance choreographers may use a guiding touch on dancers to help them achieve their specific artistic aims. Many sports and arts professionals also consider guiding touch to be a normal, traditional part of their work, as do many of their students. This may cause confusion or suspicion among outsiders, who perhaps unconsciously apply norms from civil life or appeal to a general atmosphere when assessing the practices of sports professionals (Miller et al., 2007; see Sect. 3.4). When practitioners execute specific motions in an inaccurate manner, there may be a risk that professionals providing a guiding touch will inadvertently signal a 'punishing' touch instead. On the other hand, a guiding touch may be interpreted as a sign of care, attention and professionalism by practitioners, and as such it is much appreciated (Czarnecka, 2020, p. 35).

2.1.4 Exploratory Touch

The work of some healthcare professionals, such as general practitioners, doctors and physiotherapists, inherently includes exploratory touch. Although the human body can be examined from the inside right down to the cellular level with technical devices, such devices have not completely replaced manual palpation. Indeed, palpation is often the first exploration, which is then followed by more detailed experiments. Palpating touch provides valuable information about pain in particular. The importance of exploratory touch is evident in the provision of emergency care from the outset. For example, when a caregiver inserts a drip into a patient's hand, they are already receiving essential information about the patient's condition: whether the hand is warm and dry, or cold and sweaty. By palpating the foot, one can examine whether the peripheral blood circulation is good. Pekka described the nuances of exploratory touch in his touch biography:

> I have assisted the radiologist by lifting or turning the patient after they have placed a plate under the patient for an x-ray. I have held the hand of a restless patient while the lab nurse or I have taken blood samples. I have taken the patient's blood pressure, measured their pulse and temperature. I have checked their skin. Does he have any other bruises? Is his peripheral circulation good? If their feet are unreasonably cold compared with the rest of the body, that's not a good sign. These things are only detected by touching. A 'touch patient' is typically a surgical patient. They may be bleeding or in shock etc. A patient with a fever is also a touch patient. I test it by hand – but I always tell the patient about it. (Pekka, Finnish nurse)

As the extract quoted above illustrates, exploratory touch is a concrete tool to explore and monitor the patient's overall well-being and the progress of their condition in different situations. Like all touches, exploratory touch can sometimes turn into a machine-like routine palpation. In that case, the client will probably experience it as uncomfortable—or even threatening, if it is interpreted as controlling as well. A normal reaction of the client in such a situation is to withdraw from the tactile contact, which may frustrate the professional. On the other hand, in some professional encounters the client may experience an exploratory touch as comforting. A beautician's touch is associated with luxurious pampering, but it also has an important exploratory function:

> As soon as their skin is cleansed, we tone, we blot, a quick, just over with your hands… just over the bare skin, nothing, no cleanser, nothing, so you can feel – that feels a little bit rough, that feels a bit dry, that feels a bit oily. You know, so you can feel with your bare hands what their problem is. (Welsh beautician, quoted in Straughan, 2012, p. 96)

A different investigative touch, related to security checks, is part of the normal work routines of border guards, police officers and security officers. A bodily search conducted by border authorities, police officers or prison guards is meant to ensure that the person is not carrying any weapons, illegal substances, or objects that might endanger public safety. Thus, exploratory touch has a protective function here too. In many countries, the examination may be performed only by a person of the same gender, unless it is performed by a healthcare professional. If the personal examination is directed to deeper parts of the body, under the skin, the search must be carried out in a room reserved for that purpose. Only persons of the same gender are allowed to be present when the examination extends to intimate body parts.

2.1.5 Caring and Comforting Touch

> I remember being examined on the ward of a hospital in Helsinki because of my anaemia. I had to have a sternal puncture. Even though I knew the procedure – I had assisted the doctor in such procedures several times – I was frightened. A nurse on that ward was a truly cordial and warm person. She joined the operation. When the procedure began, she took my hand and squeezed it lightly during the procedure. That touch felt good, and it reduced my fear. She didn't say anything, and I didn't say anything, but she knew I wouldn't pull my hand away – and I knew again that she was touching me with all her heart. That touch somehow gave strength. Some have this kind of skill – to approach a person correctly and sense their fears – as well as help by holding their hand. I felt like a positive heat was flowing through me. Some patients have said that I have a warm touch that is perhaps partly some kind of energy. Something undefined flows – energy. (Olga, Finnish nurse)

In her touch biography, Olga described how she had once experienced as a patient the power of a caring and supporting touch during a frightening medical treatment. She felt as if a warm energy was flowing across her own and the nurse's bodies through touch. This speaks to the affective capacities of touch. Patients who are suffering from severe disease and undergoing sometimes painful or unpleasant medical procedures reap remarkable benefits from the caring touch of professionals (e.g. Bush, 2001; Leonard & Kalman, 2015; Papathanassoglou & Mpouzika, 2012). A caring touch also relieves pain and alleviates psychophysical stress in less critical medical and nursing care situations, along a spectrum too wide to list here (see e.g. Kelly et al., 2017; Sandnes & Uhrenfeldt, 2022). Thus, as a viable, safe and cost-effective practice, caring touch has the greatest potential of the whole repertoire of professional touches, and it should be utilised systematically for the benefit of heterogeneous client types (e.g. Bush, 2001; Papathanassoglou & Mpouzika, 2012).

A caring touch may be independent of mandatory procedures and used in different encounters with the client to reinforce one's relationship with them and simply 'display some kind of humanity, warmth towards other people', as one mental health nurse expressed it (Gleeson & Higgins, 2009, p. 385). Such non-task-oriented touches may include patting or putting a hand on the client's shoulder while talking to them. Our healthcare professional interviewees mentioned holding hands as the most typical way of showing attention, care and empathy through touch and generating positive affects in their patients and clients. In this context, they often underlined the importance of 'safe areas' of the body. The upper body, particularly the arms and shoulders, were considered safe areas to touch in general, and to touch for caring purposes in particular. Gently enclosing the clients' hands in one's own strongly communicates compassion and protection to a grieving client.

Soothing touch is an important form of caring touch and may serve as an efficient tool for affect regulation (see Schlage, 2021). Many professionals in the social care, healthcare and education sectors intuitively use simple techniques of soothing touch in their daily encounters with restless children and nervous clients. Our interviews with nurses and teachers revealed that professionals perceive soothing touch to be valuable not only for individuals but also for groups of people: it can prevent fear and anxiety from spreading to other clients, thereby creating a peaceful atmosphere. It is evident that this is a very useful skill in nursery schools, for example. Soothing touch can also be used to encourage the client to gather their strength for an upcoming challenge that they fear or are nervous about. Many nurses described to us how they often felt the effects of a soothing touch on their clients corporeally: it was as if a burden was literally being lifted from the client's shoulders. 'Vilma' talked about her experiences with vulnerable older clients:

> [Touch] can start with stroking, if you want an emotional connection or to give comfort. If you brush somebody's cheek, that's obvious, you make that person smile and get eye contact. You can also see that a person enjoys it, for example, if you stroke someone's head while taking care of their hair. Yes, it evokes emotions, it is always relaxing and pleasant, and you can see in their face and gestures how the patient relaxes. (Vilma, Finnish practical nurse)

A soothing touch is especially needed before and during upsetting and frightening situations, such as medical examinations and procedures. Many clients benefit from a soothing touch in the evening before they go to bed for a restful night's sleep. Our interviewees mentioned palliative care patients and those with behavioural or memory disorders as clients who would usually benefit from a soothing touch. Such clients may be very anxious and scared, and they often seem restless and nervous. According to nursing scientist Ruth Vortherms (1991), touching that is intended to calm, support or awaken the person increases both verbal and non-verbal communication between caregivers and older adults with memory impairments. The importance of touch in dementia care was also highlighted by the care workers we interviewed. Many had found that touch led to deeper contact with people with memory problems than simply talking. Touch concretises the caregiver's attention and the intentions of care (Tanner, 2017). This is especially important given that institutional residential care contexts for the elderly and people with dementia can have dehumanising effects such as lowered self-esteem, sensory deprivation, withdrawal and depression (Bush, 2001). In addition, children and young people need a soothing touch in many situations where they are anxious, tired, irritated or sad (cf. Schneider & Patterson, 2010). 'Paula', who worked in a nursery school, stated that a soothing or encouraging touch was often a more efficient way to influence small children's affective states than spoken words:

> The fact is that through all kinds of touches you can influence affective states, you can calm or change a trouble to a joy with tickling. Touch can be so versatile. Sometimes, touch may be enough when words won't do it. (Paula, Finnish nursery schoolteacher, quoted in Keränen et al., 2017, p. 263)

Healthcare professionals may encourage the patient's family members to touch their sick or distressed loved one, for whom the touch may be crucially important (Leonard & Kalman, 2015). Rebekka, who worked on a geriatric ward, described her own approach to family members and her observations of palliative care:

> Personally, I encourage the family members to touch, and I talk about the sense of touch and how it is preserved as death approaches. Because when their loved one is at the terminal stage, a pretty typical question from them is whether the dying person knows we're here while they're sitting in the corner of the room in fear. And people usually adapt to that situation really well. And I love to see how some people go and lie side by side with the client's bed and hug tightly… But in these cases, there has usually been a really close relationship behind it, and the child has acted as the caregiver to their father… So they have already been physically so close. (Rebekka, Finnish practical nurse)

Thus, the responsibility or opportunity to provide a caring touch is not limited to professionals, even in healthcare contexts. As Rebekka's words above show, professionals can actively encourage patients and their loved ones into close physical proximity, which gives comfort and relief to both sides. However, sometimes professionals witness situations where a family member is unable even to touch their dying loved one. This often indicates a lifelong distance or severe difficulty in the relationship. On the other hand, some people fear touching their dying loved ones because they feel they may be too fragile. Further, some individuals simply do not have close relatives or other close people, and a caring touch received from professionals may be their only chance to experience emotional intimacy through touch.

Not all people have caring parents or other close persons, even as children. In her touch biography, Helka, born in 1942, recalled that she had believed during her childhood that her parents 'hated' her. Rough physical punishment was usual in her home, and she never experienced a loving touch from her parents. One day, she had a 'soul-turning' experience of caring touch. It happened in her early school years, when she hurt herself during gymnastics. The teacher rushed over to her, took her onto her lap and asked how she was. Helka burst into tears—of affection, not pain: 'I couldn't stop crying, no matter how hard I tried. […] It was more than my little heart could bear, it was a new experience'.

There are numerous nuances to the meanings that caring touch can carry, such as consolation, reassurance, encouragement and persuasion. According to nursing student Emma, a caring touch can sometimes be a 'never mind' touch, intended to alleviate the client's feelings of embarrassment or shame in delicate situations. A consoling and reassuring message is often suitable in situations where the client feels sadness, sorrow or insecurity for some reason. Sometimes, the professional may find that a touch that gives an encouraging or invigorating message is of most benefit to the client. This may be the professional's spontaneous reaction to the client's affective expressions—as is often stated regarding caring touch—but there are situations where the professional may consider an encouraging touch to be an intentional, even aggressive 'joining' with the client, a tactile alliance strategy to help them. Psychoanalyst William F. Cornell (2016) vividly describes an encounter with Adam,

2.1 Mapping Multidimensional Functions of Professional Touch   45

a young male regular client of his. When Adam initiated a handshake, Cornell responded with a firm grip on Adam's shoulders as a sign of emotional support:

> At the session's end, he stood to walk to the door, turned, put out his hand, and took my hand into a firm handshake, saying, 'See you next week.' We had never touched before. As he turned to leave, standing behind him, I reached out and placed both my hands on his shoulders in a very firm grip […]. My gesture was not spontaneous, but rather a purposive response to physically accompany Adam's reorganisation of his body toward the end of the session and his very direct way of saying goodbye and that he would be back. Here was a gesture toward the future of our work together […]. My hands on his shoulders were not acts of comfort. I was offering an aggressive contact that was a form of joining, a physical contrast to the destructive, killing anger he so much feared having within himself and showing to the world. (American psychoanalyst, Cornell, 2016, pp. 171–172.)

2.1.6 Therapeutic Touch

One important form of professional touch is therapeutic touch, by which we mainly mean complementary touch techniques that are systematically or occasionally used alongside conventional care practices and instrumental touch (e.g. Airosa et al., 2013). Although all kinds of caring touch can have therapeutic effects on the client, there are a number of techniques specifically developed for therapeutic purposes, ranging from 'classical massage' (sometimes called Swedish massage) to Rosen therapy and reiki. These techniques require special training. Experts in therapeutic touch usually operate in the private sector, but public healthcare and education professionals may also utilise these methods to promote clients' well-being. Private companies have started to develop different techniques and offer training in them in the name of therapeutic touch, and there is a qualitative richness to therapeutic touch methods—probably more so than with any other client work performed by touch.

We distinguish two main strands of therapeutic touch: (1) touching therapy systems used in massage and physiotherapy, and (2) psychotherapy-based therapeutic touch, often called 'body psychotherapy'. In classical massage and physiotherapy, the touch aims to affect the client's body, mainly on a physiological level through manipulation of the skin, fascia, muscles, tendons and vertebrae. The physiotherapist keeps a clear anatomical and physiological map in mind while manipulating the client's body. Our interviewee 'Sami', a professional masseur, explained that he used traditional massage techniques such as stroking, rubbing, squeezing, vibrating, tapping and shaking, which he adjusted to the condition and needs of each client.

The second main strand is body psychotherapy. While working, the body psychotherapist does not think of the client's body primarily through an anatomical-physiological schema. Instead, they conceive of it as an 'affective body' whereby the client's 'embodied self' is stimulated or calmed down with tactile gestures. In body psychotherapy, touch techniques involving skin contact are seen to affect the entire human nervous system, and thus touching reaches the level of the psyche. Bernhard Schlage (2021) points out that body psychotherapy aims to dissolve the dichotomy between psyche and body, and different phases of the therapy utilise different techniques, ranging from the mapping of embodied trauma to the reorganisation of the psyche. Tuula Styrman and Marika Torniainen (2018) speak of 'respectful touch' that combines multiple forms of touching, such as stroking, carrying, holding, rocking and pressing. Its purpose is to alleviate the psychophysical suffering of clients in very vulnerable states, such as convalescent patients and those living with amyotrophic lateral sclerosis.

The function of both forms of therapeutic touch is to support the client's well-being. However, body psychotherapy techniques are often included under the heading of complementary and alternative medicine. Although there is a need for further research on complementary and alternative therapies' effects on different patients, there is already evidence of their benefit from the viewpoint of subjective experience (e.g. Cheraghi et al., 2017; Henneghan & Schnyer, 2015). Some methods of therapeutic touch, such as healing energy treatments, do not actually involve any skin-to-skin contact. Nursing scientists have published studies of healing energy treatments in their scientific journals, provoking some medical scientists to critique these treatments because they lack evidence-based effects (Leskowitz, 2003; see also Cheraghi et al., 2017).

Discussing the ethics of touch in the psychotherapist's work, Marilyn Guindon and colleagues (2017) list many benefits that therapeutic touch can provide within a therapeutic relationship in the context of body psychotherapy. By exercising therapeutic touch, the therapist can (1) reorient traumatised clients and bring them back to reality, (2) calm and stabilise the autonomous nervous system and foster a sense of security, (3) help the client to explore and differentiate between aggression and pleasure, (4) deepen and balance the client's breathing, (5) maintain the client's attention and encourage them to explore their past, and (6) encourage authenticity in the therapeutic relationship and show feelings of acceptance. But although these researchers address the benefits of therapeutic touch, they also insist that these benefits are not enough in and of themselves to justify the use of therapeutic touch within the psychotherapy framework. Ethical considerations are at the heart of any exercise of touch, and in unskilled hands a therapeutic touch can turn into its opposite—an oppressive and intrusive experience for a vulnerable client.

2.1.7 Protective and Controlling Touch

By protective touch, we mean touch that prevents someone who is behaving violently or aggressively from harming themselves or others (Fredriksson, 1999, p. 1172). Protective touch may be distancing or controlling in nature. Controlling touch may be related to action-oriented contact—for example, when more than one employee is needed to restrain a client. Police officers on patrol often have to calm people who are behaving threateningly or violently in public or private places. The controlling touch may include holding a person still and leading them to a police car. It is an everyday experience for police officers to be trapped by forcible contact with a violent person. In the experience of civilians, a police officer's touch is almost always associated with some kind of negative intention, and this will be reflected in the civilian's bodily behaviour.

In medical care, protective touch is predominantly used to prevent accidents that might cause harm to patients. A patient's hand may be tied to the edge of the bed so that they cannot remove a vital device, such as an intubation tube or arterial cannula. The use of restraints is sometimes necessary in emergency care in particular, where patients may be delusional or violent. In some cases, urinary catheterisation or pad replacement is only successful if a restless or aggressive patient is held by multiple caregivers. In this kind of situation, the client naturally finds the professionals' protective touch very uncomfortable and even threatening. Although the protective and controlling touch usually restricts the client's freedom, it is justified by the intention of ensuring the patient's safety, and by the necessity to carry out some caring or medical procedure.

2.2 Merging Functions of Touch

In practical work, the boundaries between different functions are fluid and constantly transgressed, and the intentions, acts and meanings of touch are therefore highly *situational* in nature (cf. Gleeson & Higgins, 2009; Van Dongen & Elema, 2001). Mark Paterson (2004, p. 167) states that 'touch's ambiguity lies in its being active and expressive, while simultaneously being receptive and responsive'. The touched bodies react, respond and touch back in partly unpredictable ways, thereby creating a unique space-time. Erin Manning (2007) explores this idea by using Argentinian tango as a metaphor for the ambiguity of touch. Each tango is unique because the dancers can never know the exact script for their movements through touch beforehand. The boundaries of their bodies merge in their tactile movement together. Similarly, in the 'dance' between nurse and patient (cf. Kelly et al., 2017), for example, the boundaries between the worker's and patient's bodies must be flexible because of the constantly changing situation of touching (Van Dongen & Elema, 2001, p. 157).

Indeed, touch calls attention to the *relationality* of bodies and the ambivalence of the meanings and affectivities that flow across bodies, which are constantly in a state of becoming (Kinnunen & Kolehmainen, 2019). A worker who intentionally touches a client is forced to react in some way to the client's response, often by changing or diversifying the initial intention behind the touch or the kinetic manner of touching. For example, a nurse may have the intention of 'instrumentally' assisting an elderly care home resident to get dressed in the morning. But when the nurse starts to do this, the resident grasps the nurse's hand on their own and starts to cry because they miss their family. The nurse stops concentrating on getting the client dressed, sits on the bed next to the client and gives them a hug. In this situation, not only does the function of the professional's touch change, but the qualitative nuances of touch are altered as well. A connecting touch may easily merge with the comforting and encouraging functions of touch, especially during work with clients in fragile conditions or situations. Holistic tactile contact is the usual channel of communication for persons who have difficulties with verbal communication or even eye contact. Communicating through touch is also crucially important in work with the visually impaired, for example. Non-verbal cues inherently dominate some professional arenas, such as critical care, first aid and dementia care. All of these examples reveal contexts where touch seldom fulfils one clear function.

The main function of a procedural touch is to get a necessary task done. However, mandatory touch can itself also be implemented in different ways, which means that it necessarily becomes somewhat expressive and affective. For example, one might perform procedures that are frightening or (at least briefly) painful in as gentle a way as possible, or by making comforting gestures alongside the procedure. The caring and comforting function of touch should ideally be included in procedural touch whenever possible. One interviewed nursing teacher aptly illustrated the difference between 'hard' and 'soft' touches during the collection of blood samples or other procedures: 'Will you take those samples in the manner "let's keep this client still!"? Or do you take them by stroking and encouraging them?'

Indeed, we venture to suggest that caring touch should be incorporated more consciously into a wide range of necessary treatments and thus understood as a normal part of compulsory care work tasks. The nursing professionals we interviewed highlighted that some tasks—such as taking care of the client's hair, applying moisturising cream to the client's skin, and washing and shaving the client—provide natural sites for combining instrumental and caring touches. Jonna who worked in a care home talked about applying curlers in such a way as to pamper the client:

> These grandmothers for whom curlers are put in their hair, although to a lesser extent nowadays, or when their hair is being washed. The fact that you use your fingers makes them feel good… When I was a child, too, when I put curlers in my grandma's hair, it was a good moment… Here comes the touch, and they find it good when you do those things. (Jonna, Finnish practical nurse)

Although we should be wary of generalisations, older people who spend a lot of time alone often have a need to be touched by professionals (Bush, 2001). Hygiene care activities often provide practical nurses with a natural context where they can create moments of intensive presence with the client through relaxed chatting and a comforting touch. It is important to pay attention to nuances of touch during activities such as combing a client's hair or moisturising their skin. Our interviewees often mentioned a light stroking of the hair during combing, or the gentle spreading of moisturising lotion, as typical tasks that relaxed the client and encouraged them to share their inner thoughts and feelings. This of course requires a peaceful moment and a gentle orientation to the actions, even if the moment may be short. Similarly, assisting a child in daily activities, and sometimes taking the child onto one's lap, provides moments of caring and comforting touch that the child naturally needs (Schneider & Patterson, 2010). Unfortunately, the overly large groups found in nursery schools or day care often prevent professionals from providing sufficient touch for children—whose needs of course are also individual and must be discussed with parents.

2.2 Merging Functions of Touch

The touch the client receives in the beauty salon can be conceived as a procedural, comforting and therapeutic touch. The instrumental purpose of facial treatments in beauty salons is to 'deep clean' the epidermis and 'revitalise' it with masks, creams and massage. However, as ethnographic studies in Finland (Korvajärvi, 2016) and Wales (Straughan, 2012) have demonstrated, for example, cosmetologists believe that the most important function of their work is to produce tactile pleasure for their clients. The cosmetologists that Päivi Korvajärvi (2016) interviewed stressed that the most important thing in their work was to be present to their clients and offer them relaxation through the refined movements of brushing, patting, sliding and massaging. Cosmetologists themselves prefer to talk about 'pampering treatments' rather than beauty treatments.

Further, Elizabeth R. Straughan (2012) states that beauticians' touch works not only on the 'passive' surface of the face but also on the 'emotional mobilisation of the psyche or self'. The treatment provides an empathic sense of 'feeling-with', referring to the porosity of the skin: tactile contact creates a site where actions and reactions between beautician and client are mutually experienced and opened to mutual alteration. Thus, instrumental and therapeutic touches essentially merge with the comforting and connecting intentions of touch. The experience of being pampered is intensified as touch is combined with multisensory factors such as fragrant creams, aromatic oils, calming colours, soft lighting and gentle background music. More or less the same affective atmosphere can also be found in masseurs' treatment rooms, where body parts other than the head are treated.

Connecting, comforting and reassuring touches may all merge in a nurse's touch. A powerful example is provided in an account written by Nina, a young woman who participated in the project *The nurse I will never forget* in 2000. Nina had been hospitalised after a suicide attempt. She mentioned having been the object of some kind of violence, which she did not describe in detail, but which had happened before her suicide attempt. After these tragic events, she became anorexic and felt that she had 'given up forever'. While in the hospital, she felt the care personnel were distant and uninterested in knowing the real circumstances behind her tragic 'accident'. They would stop at her bedside only to complete mandatory tasks or instruct her to take her medicine. She felt like a frightened prisoner in the hospital. Then, one day, she heard a 'different footstep', which to her surprise did not simply pass by, and which was followed by a warm, 'lifesaving' touch.

> I would listen to the footsteps, and I learned to identify each walker from afar. The cautious and slightly confused footsteps of visitors, which were usually busy when they were going away. The sharp footsteps of doctors, which were always followed by critical words, orders, endless browsing of 'important' papers that were never shown to me. The ignorant footsteps of cleaners, which were always combined with the clattering of a mop handle against the edge of a bed […]. I would always close my eyes when the footsteps came closer. No matter whose they were – after all, I was just bed number three in room nine. […]
>
> Then there came some different footsteps while I was sitting on a windowsill, my back turned towards the room. I was looking at the landscape from an open window on the eleventh floor, people walking in the distance, cars, a hard asphalt courtyard onto which I might fall and everything would be over. The steps were soft, much softer than the rest, strong… and they stopped. I closed my eyes, but the steps did not continue. 'Just go', I thought. Warm

hands landed slowly on my shoulders. 'It's going to snow soon', the new arrival said, 'the last leaves are already falling, but you are not allowed to fall with them. Fight, no matter how much it hurts'. [...] I started to cry. The new arrival just put her arms around me and held me tightly but safely. For a long time, I just cried and cried, but the new arrival did not leave... they saved my life. (Nina, Finnish psychiatric patient)

2.3 Multisensory Messages

Nina's reminiscence is an impressive description of the power of multisensory communication—in this case, auditive messages combined with touch. She sensed the nurses by their footsteps' sound, rhythms and routes, and by their voices and touches. In tactile encounters, 'styles of the flesh' meet, to invoke Diane Coole's (2007) conceptualisation of face-to-face encounters. Although the context Coole describes is different—she refers mainly to conversational situations in politics—the concept of the style of the flesh can also be applied to multisensory communication in client work. According to Coole (2007, p. 425), a style is a 'relatively open, aesthetic unity of parts that has existential significance as a particular manner of being-in-the-world'. The style of the flesh consists of multisensory gestures such as vocal nuances, facial expressions, body postures, clothing and other detailed gestures and rhythms of the body. The client's experiences of touch are then intertwined with their visual, auditory, olfactory and even gustatory sensations in situations of tactile contact with the professional. These multisensory gestures comprise the client's first impression of the professional, which may have far-reaching consequences (Box 2.4).

The styles of the flesh and their rhythms may be matching or cause friction, thereby generating varied affects between the encountering bodies (Coole, 2007). Multisensory actions carry atmospheric messages—busy, intrusive and tense, or soothing, attentive and friendly, for example—and clients are tuned to respond to them in compatible ways. Imagine you have a work colleague who often rushes across the office so that you have to get out of their way. You are unlikely to feel you can stop them for a minute and tell them about your latest work ideas. Even if you do manage to stop them, if they give you an excessive handshake but avoid eye contact,

---

Box 2.4 Making a First Impression Through Bodily Gestures

Researchers have estimated that it takes between ten seconds (or less) and a few minutes to make a first physical impression, and this impression is made through one's handshake, gaze, way of speaking, body posture, and other sensory and kinetic gestures (Borg, 2013). By observing and interpreting these embodied actions, the client makes their assessment of how reliable the professional is and how easy or difficult it will be to communicate with this person in the future. A fleeting handshake is usually an easy way to convey trustworthiness, receptivity and professionalism, but sometimes its message can be the opposite. A calculated way of communicating reliability—for example, a firm handshake combined with a brisk tone of voice, rapid speech or exaggeratedly intense eye contact—can provoke suspicion and resistance in the client (see Kinnunen & Parviainen, 2016).

you will probably feel unworthy of their attention and get the message that the encounter should be kept to the minimum. The same reaction is likely from a client meeting a busy professional who does not stop to encounter them in a genuine manner. By contrast, a calm tone of voice combined with thoughtful movements will not only awaken trust and a sense of security in the client but also make it easier for the professional to reach the desired treatment goal. Indeed, it has been reported that hospital patients prefer staff to sit or bend down while communicating with them because this makes them feel noticed and secure (Edwards, 1998). By the same token, if the multisensory gestures are imbalanced, this is likely to confuse the client. A gentle touch combined with a downturned mouth or tense manner of speech may even frighten the client. But if the professional smiles and approaches the client with friendly humour, not even a limp handshake will mar the connection.

Unfortunately, the demonstration of power through touch, combined with other sensory gestures, is sometimes used to establish asymmetrical power relations or distance between a professional and a client. This can happen in several ways, but especially in the professional's way of speaking: how the professional uses words, the volume and tone of their voice, and their rhythm and intensity of speech can all strongly affect the way the client experiences and responds to the professional's touch. Some of the tasks of practical nurses are inherently difficult to perform, and they often require verbal persuasion of the client combined with gentle, secure body language and touching. The client may be receptive or may withdraw from the tactile encounter, even offending the professional in the process. The sound and tone of one's voice, the rhythm of one's movements, and other sensory gestures are important in creating an atmosphere where the client will accept mandatory measures without feeling forced into them. For a fragile person, loud speech from above and avoidant bodily gestures can feel like rough touches on the skin. An acquaintance of ours who had spent a long time undergoing cancer treatment in hospital wondered why so many nurses spoke to him in a loud voice, even though there was nothing wrong with his hearing. This type of speech, combined with their habit of bursting through the door every time they entered his room, gave him the impression that the nurses' behaviour was distancing, objectifying and impersonal, and their ostentatiously brisk speech set up a hierarchy between them and him.

Further, patting the client on the head while speaking to them in a childish tone of voice or using words that are too simple can also create an odd impression regarding the professional's intentions to connect with the client. A psychiatrist we know, a man in his 70s, told us about his outrageous experience as a patient on a hospital ward. Many of the nurses talked to him and his roommate, a retired army officer, as if they were little children. They found this hard to take, and they could not decide whether it was flattering or humiliating. A study conducted in the US investigated people's experiences of being touched by nurses while in hospital (O'Lynn & Krautscheid, 2011). The participants expected professionalism and respect from the staff, and they felt this was contravened when staff were overfamiliar. For example, they felt annoyed if a nurse addressed them as 'we' ('how are we today?') or 'honey', used their first name without asking permission, or did not look them in the eye and/or talked to other nurses while performing hygiene care tasks.

The behaviours just described—distancing on one hand, overfamiliar on the other—probably do not (or not often) arise from a conscious intention to humiliate clients. More likely, they are tacitly learned patterns of 'normal' communication with clients in the work community. In any case, overly distancing bodily practices, as well as notably ambivalent sensory gestures, can damage the most vulnerable patients, and this must be taken seriously. To judge from stories we have heard from patients and professionals alike, it is far too common for patients in psychiatric hospitals in particular to encounter humiliating and potentially damaging behaviours.

2.4 Styles and Techniques of Professional Touch

From the angle of a client, *all* touches are affectively charged or emotionally expressive because even the simplest procedures are carried out by some style of touching. It has been reported that patients can recognise individual nurses from their specific touch styles, even if they have no other way of knowing who the toucher is (Routasalo, 1997, p. 295). 'Sofia' who worked on a long-term care unit told us during her interview that one of her visually impaired clients could recognise her from her touch style. This client also responded to her touch in an individualised manner, differently from the way the client interacted with other nurses. Our interviewee found her unique tactile communication with this client professionally rewarding because she interpreted it as a sign that she had successfully created a connection with the patient. In everyday life, tactile metaphors are used to describe whole persons: some people are said to be 'soft' or 'warm', while others may be known as 'rough' or 'cold' (cf. Van Dongen & Elema, 2001, p. 152). No doubt, this applies to encounters with professionals, of whose personalities clients make comprehensive assessments by virtue of their touching styles and other sensory gestures.

Clients register different professionals' touch styles through nuances, which can be both extremely rich and systematically developed (Box 2.5). The touch of a professional may feel pleasant or uncomfortable, soothing or distressing, safe or unsafe, even though we can seldom specify the exact reasons why. These feelings are immediately stored in the body's memory when we experience them. Based on our findings from various research materials, we conclude that clients categorise touching styles through the following rough dichotomies:

distant/close
harsh/smooth
firm/tentative
hostile/kind
fast/slow
absent/present
insecure/secure
unidirectional/bidirectional
neutral/affective

> **Box 2.5 Hapteces and Haptemes**
> The subtlety of meaning that nuanced touching can convey is specifically important for people with visual impairments or deafblindness. According to Riitta Lahtinen's (2008) analysis, this communication happens through 'hapteces', which consist of touches of different qualities and dimensions ('haptemes'). The haptemes include the duration, location, intensity, extent, frequency of repetition, and number of repetitions of touch. Thus, hapteces are made up of haptemes insofar as we recognise tactile haptemes as direction of movement, change of direction on the body, pressure, speed, frequency, size, length, duration, pause, change of rhythm, shape, and macro and micro movements. Simple hapteces may be one's only form of communication when working with people with dementia, since 'touch pervades all aspects of dementia care', as Cristina Douglas (2021) states based on her ethnographic fieldwork in Scottish dementia care facilities. Douglas says that touch is a channel in daily actions through which to form the vitally important connection between client and carer, who become intimately entangled through touch as a condition of living.
>
> Haptemes play a crucial role in work with people with severe developmental disabilities, young children, and people in end-of-life care. Haptemes also convey important information in the training of instrumentalists and vocalists, and in athlete coaching. Haptemes are a natural part of the working methods of physiotherapy too. For example, a physiotherapist may put their hand on a client's shoulder to give them a signal to stop and calm down. If the physiotherapist adds a new hapteme to the same touch, such as a small pull backwards, it may signal to the touched person that they should move backwards.

withdrawn/dialogic
predetermined/spontaneous
controlled/ambivalent
serious/playful

Our interviewees often used thermal words to determine pleasant and unpleasant touches. For example, Sofia told us about a colleague of hers who had received positive feedback for her 'warm hands'. With those hands the colleague could create the feeling of safety, including for 'more difficult' clients so that they would not 'fight back'—a reference to clients with dementia or Alzheimer's disease, who can behave unpredictably during care procedures. By 'warm hands', Sofia meant the specific energy and affectivity her colleague's hands transmitted to clients. As a general rule, if you wish to create a pleasant touch, Sofia suggested, 'you can't grab the patient in your cold fingers but softly with your whole warm hands'. This comment about 'cold fingers' echoed a well-known fact that is also confirmed by several studies: an unpredictable and rough touch performed by cold hands is the most unpleasant of all professional touches. Sofia referred to her own hands as 'innately cold', by which she meant their literal physical temperature rather than her style of touching.

Therefore, she would touch the patient's hand or cheek first, as if to warn them about her cold fingers before beginning the actual procedure.

Sofia's reference to the 'whole hands' also encompassed a firmness of touch, which she considered especially important to minimise any potential hurt from the touch 'when there is a lot of bone surface to be touched in the patient's body'. It is evident that the general conception among healthcare professionals is that the correct grip should be 'firm but still gentle', as many characterised it. Several professionals, from nurses to personal trainers, stressed that a touch that was 'too light', 'fumbling', 'insecure' or 'hesitant' would immediately arouse distrust in the client and impede the work. On the affective level, such a touch might fail to convey a message of care and empathy to the client, instead giving an impression of uncertainty and insecurity. On the other hand, 'too rough' a touch might be experienced as an assault. The interviewees also stated that a firm grip was extremely important when one is touching a person whose legs no longer bear their weight. Moving from one place to another will feel frightening to the client if the grip exudes a lack of experience, or insecurity for some other reason. In addition, with the performance of position management for patients in palliative care in particular, our interviewees emphasised the importance of a firm but delicate touch to make the turns as safe, comfortable and painless as possible.

Besides the different qualities of one's grip, one's professional touch style is determined by the time spent touching (O'Lynn & Krautscheid, 2011). A nurse who worked on a long-term care unit commented on different touch styles by saying 'some of us are faster and others slower'. Like nurses in general, she seemed to believe that 'being slow' is inherently better than 'being fast'—which to a great extent of course is a matter not just of personal touch style but also external working conditions. However, from an objective point of view, providing a caring touch does not necessarily require many 'extra' minutes; rather, it is about 'stretching time' through touch, to evoke Styrman and Torniainen (2018), the developers of the method of 'respectful touch' (see Sect. 2.1.6). Styrman and Torniainen claim that investing in just a few seconds of thoughtful touch can work miracles. Ideally, all touches in care work should be performed by 'landing' the hands calmly and softly on the client's skin, Styrman and Torniainen advise. Indeed, several studies have already demonstrated that even a brief but unhurried moment of caring touch—in early childhood services, schools, hospitals or care homes, for example—may be of unexpected value to a child or adult client (e.g. Connor & Howett, 2009; Dobson et al., 2002; Field, 2003; Kelly et al., 2017; Lindgren et al., 2014; Schneider & Patterson, 2010). A home care worker we interviewed also discussed this topic. She said that putting a hand on a client's shoulder when one was about to leave their home did not take much time but delivered an impressive improvement in the client's mental well-being, at least temporarily. Another healthcare professional stressed that even the smallest 'extra' moment of unhurried time 'repays itself a hundredfold'.

Explanations for touch styles extend from psychological personality theories to views about cultural learning. Psychological studies of the use of touch in management and workplace behaviour state that touch is an effective channel of communication for people with high self-esteem. Based on their own experimental studies, an American team of management researchers state that when touch is used in appropriate ways in the workplace, it generates positive responses among coworkers, including trust in the support, sincerity, care and likeability of the initiator of the touch (Fuller et al., 2011). Touch can also play an important role in apologies and forgiveness. In general, it is a powerful means to enhance the effectiveness of interpersonal communication for those with 'touch self-efficacy', i.e. those who believe in their own ability to communicate actively and properly through touch in a work context. However, the researchers also point out that the touch initiator's self-esteem is not the only factor in the outcomes of touching. Cultural backgrounds, workplace norms, gender, personal needs, and the interpretation and type of touch are some of the factors that contribute to actual experiences of touch (Fuller et al., 2011). These factors are tied to a great extent to socialisation processes and situational variables, as we stress throughout this book.

Socialisation to professional touch occurs to a great extent via professional education and work institutions, whether situated in the public or private sector. Our acting as part of a collegial society deeply influences the way we construct our professional identities and the working methods we adopt, and this happens largely unconsciously. Researchers use the concept of the organisational body (e.g. Hassard et al., 2000) to refer to the ways in which employees' bodies are socialised into shared practices, norms and values, and even into feeling rules and ways to 'manage heart and mind' (Hochschild, 1983). Adopting normative touch practices is an essential part of acquiring the desired organisational body, although it is often only newcomers who so much as recognise the existence of a specific touch culture—long-term employees tend to take practices for granted. Tanner (2017) distinguishes between *task-centred* and *person-centred* organisational cultures in dementia care. Task-centred organisational cultures maintain professional boundaries by keeping clients at a distance and avoiding emotional intimacy. With regard to touch practices, staff members in such cultures are most worried about cynical accusations from outsiders, and they therefore concentrate on protecting themselves. Affectionate touch is a taboo in this type of organisational culture. In person-centred cultures, however, providing an affectionate touch when necessary is a natural part of working practice. As Tanner (2017, pp. 53–54) reminds us, touch styles convey messages about the relationship between client and professional, whether those styles be:

loving/hostile
encouraging/restraining
supportive/undermining
calming/distressing
comforting/agitating
warm/cold
gentle/harsh
tender/unfeeling

personal/objectifying
close/distant
caring/controlling
kind/aggressive

Experimental studies have demonstrated that touch alone can effectively communicate various elementary emotions—anger, fear, happiness, sadness, disgust, love, gratitude, sympathy—between two strangers. In one such study, psychologists arranged a test where an 'encoder' was asked to communicate the above-mentioned emotions to a 'decoder' by touching them in the manner they deemed correct on the appropriate body parts. The decoder was asked to interpret the communicated emotions. The members of these dyads could not see or hear each other, and they communicated only through a hole in a barrier. Several types of tactile stimulus were used in the experiment, including squeezing, stroking, rubbing, pushing, pulling, pressing, patting, tapping, shaking, pinching, vibrating, poking, hitting, scratching, massaging, tickling, slapping, hugging, interlocking (of fingers), swinging and throwing. The decoders drew distinctions between all these tactile movements and their intensity and duration. The finding of the experiment was that touch is an even more nuanced way to communicate different positive and negative emotions than facial or vocal expressions (Hertenstein et al., 2009). This particular study was conducted in the US, but it is probable that the key argument applies to most cultures, including professional organisational cultures: touch is a powerful vehicle for expressing nuanced emotions and transmitting affects across bodies.

The professional's level of experience naturally influences their touch style. For example, a newly qualified nurse or early childhood educator may touch insecurely or hesitantly, whereas an experienced professional's grip will exude routinised confidence. One's presence or absence through touch, on the other hand, does not depend on the length of one's work experience. Some nursing students we interviewed said they had observed that newcomers still had the energy to pay attention to their style of touch and were ready to provide 'something extra' to the client besides the necessary procedures. Previous research has also made the same finding (Dobson et al., 2002). Our interviewees frowned upon older colleagues who 'confine themselves to mechanically conducting only the minimum', a problem they encountered all too often. On the other hand, however, the most experienced nurses we interviewed had observed precisely the opposite: newly qualified nurses rushed their tasks and then hurried back home. We conclude that there is no reason to generalise about either group.

Organisational cultures are constantly in the making, and new practices emerge. Touch itself is a 'fundamental medium of the expression, experience and contestation of social values and hierarchies', as Constance Classen (2005, p. 1) reminds us. For example, the practical nurse Sari described how she had changed her general conception of professional touch over the course of her decades-long career. She said that she was always learning more, especially about the expressive and therapeutic functions of touch, although the organisation itself had never really addressed this in training, meetings etc. However, along with her constant learning, she was able to renew the practices of her collegial institution. Many of the professionals we interviewed also realised that their own touch styles arose not only from shared workplace practices but also from their personal backgrounds. Thanks to their lifelong personal experiences of touch, some professionals may accept touch as a natural part of their working method, while others may experience it as strange or even unpleasant (Sect. 3.1). We agree with Coole (2007, pp. 425–426) that 'styles of the flesh' are deep-rooted structures that offer limited scope for improvisation. However, the main point of this book as a whole is that if one is conscious of one's own and other people's corporeal styles and their potential origins and effects, one can learn to improvise too. Touch inevitably conveys the professional's emotions and moral attitudes, and also evokes them in the client's body.

In one brief moment of touching, a whole organisation's values and practices can also be expressed through the professional's style of communication. But shared practices of touch matter not only because of corporate image, but also for very practical reasons. For example, severely weak patients are often cared for by pairs or small teams of nurses, whose mutual corporeal working styles must be in harmony. The nurses in such cases have to coordinate their actions and produce 'intercorporeal ways of knowing' and acting through routines, while simultaneously adapting each move to the situation at hand (see Hindmarsh & Pilnick, 2007). 'Liisa', who worked on a psychogeriatric ward, told us that such seamless intercorporeal work might even help to cut staffing costs:

> I know, since I have been working here right from the beginning and been working with a smaller team. We are four nurses who have also gone elsewhere to train colleagues in how to approach clients with behavioural disorders in different situations. I am quite sure that if there are like-minded people on a working team, there will be no need for more care personnel. And the work tasks will be done as effectively, and there will be no major conflicts if people are just like-minded. (Liisa, Finnish practical nurse)

The healthcare professionals we interviewed stressed that whatever an individual's touch style may be, it should always convey a message of respect and signal an awareness of the client's condition and personal background, if known. Further, touch should give the impression that the client is important and equal, and that their private space is respected (see also Gleeson & Higgins, 2009). Of course, the proper style and technique depend on the profession. In surveillance and front-line police work, touch is usually involved in work tasks in situations where there is a risk of violence or a need to use physical force. Touch is also the working tool of beauticians and masseurs, albeit in entirely the opposite way to police work. No one is likely to assume that police officers should touch citizens in the same way as beauticians touch their clients. Confusing situations may arise if the professional's touch style diverges dramatically from the client's expectations of professional touch. In order for a professional to understand and develop their own touch style, it is extremely important for them to recognise their personal relationship with touch—the experiences, capacities, potentialities, learned habits and affective repertoires attached to touch (Sect. 3.1). This will help the professional to catch the intercorporeal 'vibrations' and meaning-makings that emerge in touch with the client: how do I interpret the client's feelings, why do I feel like this, what is happening between us?

2.5 Managing one's Own Affects and Emotions

One aspect of using touch to fulfil one's duties at work is that all forms of professional touch generate affects in the professional's own body. The skilful use of touch often generates emotionally rewarding experiences for the professional who feels they have acted in ethically sustainable ways and succeeded in helping the client (Sect. 5.8). Caring touch in particular can be perceived as a concrete act that is permeated by feelings of goodwill towards the client. In work contexts, caring touch differs from loving touch, which does not fall within the scope of professional touch—although female teachers, for example, often compare their way of touching children to 'mothering' them (Estola, 2003; Kinnunen & Seppänen, 2009). However, in caring touch, the professional does express feelings of affection, empathy and goodwill to enhance the client's psychophysical condition. Instead of being a superficial gesture practised beforehand, caring touch has been described as spontaneous, unselfish and therapeutic by nature (e.g. Chang, 2001; Fredriksson, 1999). Many of our nurse interviewees seemed to believe that clients could tell whether a nurse was really present and caring or was only pretending. A middle-aged female cancer patient commented on this by reflecting on her doubts about the genuineness of the emotion behind the nurses' touch:

> They'll touch you and say, you know, 'I'm sorry about this, and you'll get through it.' And that touch is supposed to be reassuring, I think. But it's, to me, it's more like, I wasn't offended, but it was token… It was all part of the medical procedure… It wasn't like a personal touch. Their brains aren't even involved in the touch. (North American patient, quoted in Leonard & Kalman, 2015, p. 519)

The tension between 'deep feeling' and 'surface feeling' is always present in client work in some way, as Arlie Hochschild (1983) concluded. Although clients expect service providers to bring their genuine personalities to work, workers need to protect themselves from the depth of their own emotions and to distance themselves from the client relationship. This demands conscious and constant training in emotion management. In her fieldwork with care workers in US hospices, Cindy L. Cain (2017) found that certain feeling rules pertained to caring work, including emotion management skills: listening, truly caring, keeping calm and maintaining boundaries. The latter is often believed to be hard to learn, especially for female workers. Here lies the paradox of emotional work: how can one be genuinely present and honestly feel empathy for the client while simultaneously protecting oneself from deep, exhausting feelings? As a professional, how can one learn to distance oneself from certain stressful situations without harming the client? We believe that all forms of professional touch can be consciously developed without leading to emotional overload or ethically dubious practices—a topic we consider in more depth in Chap. 5.

2.5 Managing one's Own Affects and Emotions

Sometimes, touching a client can give rise in a professional to 'forbidden' feelings towards the client. For example, while performing necessary tasks related to the client's hygiene, or in the context of controlling or protective touch, professionals may feel confusion, shame, disgust, fear, anger or excitement, which they will often perceive as unprofessional and inappropriate, and which they think they must hide not only from the client but also from their colleagues (cf. Van Dongen & Elema, 2001). In such situations, affective work means aiming for as neutral a touching style as possible and suppressing one's own affects in order to protect the client's feelings. It is important that touch and other sensory gestures should not convey any negative affects to the client, regardless of how the professional themselves experiences the touch (and leakages) of the cared-for body. In his touch autobiography, Pekka described his uncomfortable feelings in challenging situations, particularly on the emergency unit:

> If you find some touch unpleasant, you should not show it. You just have to keep it in your mind – it is not allowed to be visible in your face or heard in your voice… Situations in which I feel uncomfortable can be like the following. The patient is dirty, untidy and smells bad, is drunk and cantankerous. Then I try to perform the touch as quickly as possible and using gloves. Gloves are like little shield – 'I wanna keep a distance from you, and I'm doing this only because I have to'… Gloves are used quite a lot today, even if the patient is not dirty. It is a question of hygiene. A touch with a glove is somehow more distant… it becomes more 'sterile'.
>
> Incidents of violence are also tiresome. You often face this problem in emergency care. The patient may scratch, squeeze your arm, suddenly hit you, grab your hair etc. Over twenty-five years I was forced to face these too. Of course, you don't even think about these occasions and don't even want to remember them. The patient may have been on crack or having psychotic symptoms. Such occasions have increased my own attentiveness, but bad things still happen. They haven't traumatised me anyhow, and I don't even remember their names or how they looked. However, you remember a kick or punch for a long time. Also, verbal insults were commonplace. Fortunately, then you don't have to touch. If the patient is totally disoriented and dangerous to themselves or others, the doctor has the right to order restraints… Sometimes, you are forced to put a mask over the patient's mouth if they spit. (Pekka, Finnish nurse)

This extract demonstrates that a professional may resort to gloves or other accessories and means, not only to protect themselves from infection, but also to distance themselves from direct skin contact with the client, which in turn protects them emotionally. It also illustrates typical situations where the professional has to rely on a protective or controlling touch, the affective reactions that can arise in the professional's body following such situations, and the difficulties one might face when attempting to process one's own affects 'professionally'. Pekka experienced ambivalence between 'professional' and 'private' feelings when faced with a violent client, an ambivalence to which one of us authors can also relate. Over 20 years ago, Taina Kinnunen worked in a children's home, and one morning she experienced a sudden aggressive attack by a teenager. Taina had entered the home and was just about to start the morning shift when she encountered a resident who was apparently in a confused state after having used drugs the night before. When Taina asked the girl to get on with her morning activities, the girl suddenly grabbed Taina's hair, pulling it violently and shouting at the same time. The girl's voice and gaze were full of anger and anxiety. In that situation, Taina saw no other way to ensure the client's and her own security than to grab the girl around the upper body and press her forcefully against a wall until she calmed down.

The incident left far-reaching marks on Taina's embodied memory. She felt she had been wounded not only physically but above all psychically. It took her a long time to get over what had happened, perhaps partly because she had received no preparation at all for this kind of incident during her youth work training. She realised immediately after the attack that there had not been a single word on the curriculum about professional touch or what to do in situations of violence. She also felt sorry for the girl, who seemed confused and ashamed after the attack but could not really deal with it. Thus, Pekka and Taina shared the same embarrassment, caused by the ambiguity that arises when one's professional self says, 'I don't mind, it's part of the job' while the private self says, 'I can't help feeling wounded'.

In some situations, a protective and controlling touch may be the only solution to ease the tension, even though it often leaves clients and nurses alike with a 'bad feeling' (Estabrooks, 1989). Researchers have found that healthcare professionals may use blocking tactics, avoidance and distancing if they are afraid of losing control over an extremely stressful situation (Connor & Howett, 2009). Sometimes the avoidance of touch is the most protective available practice regarding not only physical security but also the professional's emotional resources. For example, teachers may need to protect themselves from the emotions that arise when faced with a child who is suffering mistreatment. In such situations, the teacher may avoid using comforting touch and seek instead to resolve the situation through constructive, 'rational' discussion with the child's parents. Another mechanism that professionals may use to protect themselves emotionally is to discharge their own frustration through negative or aggressive touch. For example, security guards or bouncers may use a rough controlling touch in situations where they have not been able to alleviate the tension by any positive means. In these jobs, as well as in police work, the decision to act physically must often be taken in seconds, with no time to consider the alternatives or to sufficiently adjust the quality of the touch to protect oneself or others. Of course, it is also possible that professionals sometimes take advantage of their own position of power and intentionally use hard grips on clients in an unethical way.

At the end of the working day, police officers, nurses and beauticians put down their duties and roles, detach themselves from professional manners of touch, and again become husbands, mothers, grandfathers, daughters, friends and neighbours. The transition is not always fully successful, since the bodily practices created at work may also be reflected in everyday relationships and leisure activities. In some cases too, such as police officers, a heightened awareness of certain professional practices and ethics is expected to be maintained outside working hours. Therefore, the professional's 'civil personality' cannot and should not be completely detached from their work identity, as we have stressed. This in turn makes 'professional touch' partly inaccessible to concepts and theories.

As human beings, all professionals carry emotional loads that are unrelated to their encounters at work but easily come to resonate with them. Therefore, although affective work is to a certain extent done through one's own body and touch, it is necessary to be able to separate one's working self from one's private self. 'Hanna', who worked as a nurse in sheltered housing, described how her bus journey between work and home, and the change of clothes at either end, were ritualistic transitions between her professional and private selves. When she was dressed in her nurse's uniform, she felt ready to encounter her patients professionally. Another nurse, 'Merja', described in her touch biography that her 'overly empathic and omniscient' professional role was replaced by her civil self at the end of the shift. When she boarded the bus home, she sometimes even found the physical proximity of strangers 'tiresome', unlike at work. Her civil self wanted to touch only the people she loved.

2.6 Listening to the Client

> I think that the person must be approached holistically, what is there in the background? And what different forms of touch include: how hard or lightly I can touch. Of course, you have to consider sexuality, gender and so on. My opinion is that professional touch should cover a consciousness of all these, one way or another. (Iida, Finnish nursing student)

> I must stop in front of that person. I must think for a while what aims do we have, what kind of situation do we have here? What are we doing, and where are we going? […] Depends on the person. […] Quite often it is not just the touch but expressions, gestures and everything else. But if it is quiet so that you can take your time without hurrying, the outcome is good. (Kaisa, Finnish practical nurse)

In a client-oriented encounter, the professional genuinely aims to understand how the client prefers to be touched, and whether it is justified to minimise tactile contact. Some clients may experience a professional's touch as embarrassing or even threatening if they have had previous experience of violence or abuse, for example. A person with dementia may resist—perhaps even violently—necessary procedures that target intimate body parts, behaviour which some of our nurse interviewees thought might sometimes be explained by traumatic experiences in the person's past (see also Dobson et al., 2002). There are also clients for whom all touches are painful, at least in some situations. On the other hand, some clients have an exceptional need for the professional's attention through touch in order to feel safe. Clients also differ in their receptiveness to and preferences for different touch styles. Some prefer a light and others a tight grip; some cannot stand quick movements, while others appreciate them. Most clients probably expect the professional to manage all these nuances in their proper contexts, which can sometimes be challenging. One nurse interviewee put it like this: 'It is a kind of eternal question whether the touch grip is gentle enough while remaining tight'. Many interviewees seemed to think that professional touch is all about the ability to utilise the power and quality of touch in proper ways, according to each client and their specific condition and needs.

Professionals touch clients in their professional roles, which are regulated by legal guidelines and professional codes of ethics (Sect. 1.5). At the same time, a tactile encounter is a negotiation and reconciliation between two individuals, each of whom has a unique personal and cultural background that is embodied in their touch style. The client's style of the flesh and their manner of touch should be the starting point for the choreography of the encounter. The healthcare professionals and students we interviewed had a lot to say about the importance of 'sensing', 'listening to' or 'reading' the client. Most of them could not describe in detail how they did this themselves. 'You just learn it through experience' or 'you can see it immediately from the client's posture and appearance' were typical ways to describe their intuitive knowledge of how to touch and approach clients in general.

Emma, a nursing student specialising in gerontology and medical and surgical nursing, emphasised that the professional needed to know the right way before touching the client rather than afterwards, because touching in the 'wrong' way could immediately ruin their chances of building a trusting relationship. Kaisa, who worked as a practical nurse, stated that the client should be delicately 'invited' to touch by sensitive, tentative gestures. However, there were often procedures that simply had to be done, and in these situations Kaisa could forget that the client might feel embarrassed or irritated even though Kaisa herself regarded touch as a self-evident working method. On the other hand, previous studies have noted that nurses learn to rely on their own observations of patients' body language to establish whether a patient is comfortable with touch (see also Sect. 3.5). In a study conducted in Ireland (Gleeson & Higgins, 2009), psychiatric nurses said they let the patients initiate the most 'intimate' touches, such as kissing and embracing, and would only respond reciprocally thereafter. They explained that they would 'honour their client's personal space' by default if the client was unknown to them, was experiencing psychosis or came from a different cultural background. These nurses stressed that patients' verbal and non-verbal cues were informative, as did our interviewees too:

> Even just touching their hand, you'll know if somebody is going to pull away. If they feel uncomfortable then you've crossed a boundary. You'll get verbal and non-verbal cues off patients if you've entered their personal space, if they're recoiling from you. (Irish psychiatric nurse, quoted in Gleeson & Higgins, 2009, p. 386)

Care professionals sometimes face problematic situations if a patient is very frail and cannot speak, and they must then find the proper way to communicate with them. Even in such situations, touch may well not be the primary way of providing attention and care to the patient:

> A family member has told me that the client has never liked to be pawed – has used that word. Well, then – how can you provide relaxation and sort of pleasure? For example, if massaging their hands or feet does not feel good, what might it be then? What might reach a person who cannot speak any more? That's really something to think about. (Tyyne, Finnish nurse)

When it comes to touch, every professional is naturally expected to respect the client's wishes as far as possible in all situations. However, touch itself may often be the most fruitful channel to gain valuable information about the client's condition, to sense their physical and emotional state, and then to act accordingly. Sami, the masseur we interviewed, described how a client's handshake, gait, facial expression and way of speaking all revealed something about the client's psychophysical condition and social situation, even before the massage began. Palpating the client's body parts during the massage was his last clue as to whether to manipulate their muscles delicately or with a tight grip. Sami felt the degree of tension in the client's body through touch, which informed him about the client's overall condition. By 'listening' to the client's body through his hands, he tried to choose the right technique to respond to the client's psychophysical state. It was not a matter of simply choosing a tight grip with a tense client or a gentle touch with a relaxed client, rather the opposite, in fact. When a person's body is prima facie very troubled, it should not be further troubled by the masseur's touch, Sami stressed.

As a working skill, touching easily falls into the category called 'soft skills', which includes multiple social skills such as listening, negotiation, communication, persuasion, presentation and reading body language. These skills cannot be detached from one's own embodied personality, attitude, flexibility, style and motivation. As a smooth, embodied skill, touching seems to run more or less on its own—to be immune to external influence (at least when all is going well). But we argue that when coping with uncertain work environments, people need to foster (pre)reflective attitudes and to be open to more subtle and indirect influences. Thus, one should resist the type of automation that phenomenologist Herbert Dreyfus (2002; Dreyfus & Dreyfus, 1986) ascribes to the highest levels of expertise where embodied skills are based on neither thinking nor awareness, neither attention nor choice, at the level of fluid performance.

Instead, we stress that although touch skills may be part of the embodiment of expertise, professionals need to become and remain aware of those skills in order to practise and cultivate them. We refer to Elizabeth Ennen's (2003) formulations of 'skill memory' and 'habit memory' to emphasise the reflective fluidity of using touch during expert activity. Ennen emphasises that skill memory and habit memory are two different things. Skill memory refers to the acquisition of a capacity to perform a sequence of movements fluidly and automatically; habit memory is the acquisition of a disposition to respond automatically to a particular stimulus. Grounded in non-representational mechanisms, touching *as a combination of skill memory and habit memory* is highly context-dependent, responding readily in complex but specific ways. Ideally, the open-ended and flexible performance of the touching act will be context-sensitive, and it will respond sensitively to subtle changes in the situation. Such smooth and unobtrusive responsiveness to circumstances is reflective in nature, but it does not require any conscious knitting together of distinct sensations, such as tactile sensations of surfaces or kinaesthetic sensations of bodily movement. For these reasons, reflective responses based on the skill memory of touching are fast and fluid—quite unlike the slow, conscious decision-making processes that draw explicitly on declarative knowledge (Sutton et al., 2011).

Professional touching has aptly been called an 'art and skill' that combines tacit and rational knowledge and requires constant improvisation according to the changing situation. In the context of nursing, Van Dongen and Elema (2001, p. 150) state: 'Tacit knowledge is based on experience of nursing and intuition, rapid and goal-oriented. Rational knowledge can be obtained by education'. Based on their own participant observation in psychiatric care settings in the Netherlands, they conclude that nurses move between the 'objectification' and 'subjectification' of their own and their patients' bodies. We agree, and we would add that nurses (and other professionals) balance between distant and close, neutral and affective touching. A skilful professional is able to adapt their touching style to ongoing situations with different clients of varied backgrounds and acute needs. This makes their touching style an artistic practice whose importance is even more crucial in multicultural environments:

> Touching as an art means that people have to redefine, reinvent and reshape their ways of touching others day by day, situation by situation. That touch is an 'uncertain' activity that needs constant listening to the body is all the more clear in a multicultural society where people live together with different systems of touching. (Van Dongen & Elema, 2001, p. 153)

Of course, professional touch as the art of improvising according to changing situations and unpredictable events should not be understood merely as an individual skill. Rather, it is dependent on work circumstances, which are often extremely demanding. As Rachel Lara Cohen (2011, p. 196) states, bodies have their own material rhythms and processes, and this makes all types of body work impossible to predict precisely. We also stress that this should always be taken into account when one is thinking about touch: it is impossible to predict the kinds of touch that will be needed with different patients in different situations. People's emotions and affective states are also partly unpredictable processes.

2.7 Thematic Learning Tasks

2.7.1 Reflection Activities

1. Think about a normal working day in your own job, or perhaps in an internship related to your future profession. Consider the following questions:
   - What different functions of professional touch (connecting touch, procedural touch etc.) can you identify in your work performance?
   - Do you find some forms of professional touch more pleasant and inspiring than others?
   - Which touch practices cause you anxiety or stress?
2. Choose one function of professional touch that is highly typical of the organisation where you work (e.g. connecting touch or procedural touch):
   - Can you recognise differences in personal style among your colleagues?
   - Does your organisation have common and shared touch practices that everyone follows?
   - If there are shared touch practices, how do they convey the whole organisation's cultural values?
3. Put yourself in the client's shoes and recollect your own tactile encounters with professionals in client work sectors. Choose one pleasant encounter to reflect on:
   - Why did that encounter through touch feel pleasant and comfortable?
   - Were you able to register the professional's emotions, affective state and moral attitudes?
   - How did this encounter differ from your unpleasant experiences of professional touch?

2.7 Thematic Learning Tasks

4. Think about the new insights and learnings with which this chapter has provided you:
   - What skills and competences do you already have—perhaps without having recognised them before—in the forms of professional touch?
   - What weaknesses or limitations can you identify in your habitual touch that you might develop further?
   - What support would you need, and from whom, for this development?

2.7.2 Fieldwork

Touch is a powerful vehicle for expressing emotions and transmitting affects across bodies. There have been efforts to identify touch styles and different qualities of touch, but so far little is known about how professionals are able to transmit complex information through touch. You can advance this knowledge by conducting a little autoethnographic fieldwork. Ask one of your colleagues to perform some of their typical tactile working tasks on you. Tell them that this experiment is related to your studies and this textbook. You can write notes about your observations, impressions and feelings later, and you can also discuss the experience with your participating colleague. Focus on the affects and information transmitted through touch during the experiment. The following questions may help you with your ethnographic report:

- How would you describe the events during the touch situation and the atmosphere of the encounter (e.g. was it tense or relaxed)?
- Try to describe as accurately as possible how you experienced the touch and skin contact in this encounter. Was there any technology-mediated touch? How did that feel?
- What were your colleague's thoughts, intentions, experiences and observations of the situation? Compare your own and your colleague's interpretations.

2.7.3 Case Study

Return to Sect. 2.1.1 and the example of the Finnish nurse who had worked in Saudi Arabia. Reread the description and think about any cultural differences you have noticed in your own life or work career—e.g. closeness and distance in connecting touch. In his touch biography, the nurse wrote about his experiences in the following way:

> I shook hands with the patients' male family members as much as five times a day. They could come within thirty centimetres of me, touch my shoulder or chest. You soon get used to that anyway – you must respect their way. A grateful patient or family member could even kiss my cheek or forehead, the way they greet good friends, relatives or respected persons. As such, there was of course nothing sexual in their touch. It was only cultural etiquette. A hand on my shoulder told me that he respects me. A hand on my chest meant that he respects me both as a person and as a nurse and trusts me – and leaves his loved ones in my care.

- What distance do you consider appropriate or comfortable when you are greeting clients, and when do you feel that the client is too far away from you, or too close? How do you respond in these situations?
- What cultural differences have you noticed in the way clients greet you by touching?
- Does the client's gender or age affect how you greet or otherwise touch them in your work tasks? If so, how did you come to touch them differently?

References

Airosa, F., Falkenberg, T., Öhlén, G., & Arman, M. (2013). Tactile massage or healing touch: Caring touch for patients in emergency care – A qualitative study. *European Journal of Integrative Medicine, 5*(4), 374–381.

Borg, J. (2013). *Body language. How to know what's REALLY being said*. Pearson.

Bush, E. (2001). The use of human touch to improve the well-being of older adults: A holistic nursing intervention. *Journal of Holistic Nursing, 19*(3), 256–270.

Cain, C. L. (2017). Boundaried caring and gendered emotion management in hospice work. *Gender, Work and Organization, 24*(4), 345–359.

Camps, J., Tuteleers, C., Stouten, J., & Nelissen, J. (2013). A situational touch: How touch affects people's decision behavior. *Social Influence, 8*(4), 237–250. https://doi.org/10.1080/15534510.2012.719479

Chang, S. O. (2001). The conceptual structure of physical touch in caring. *Journal of Advanced Nursing, 33*(6), 8210–8827.

Chang, E. S., & Levy, B. R. (2021). High prevalence of elder abuse during the COVID-19 pandemic: Risk and resilience factors. *The American Journal of Geriatric Psychiatry, 29*, 1152–1159. https://doi.org/10.1016/j.jagp.2021.01.007. Epub 2021 Jan 19. PMID: 33518464; PMCID: PMC8286979.

Cheraghi, M. A., Sadat Hosseini, A. S., Gholami, R., Bagheri, I., Binaee, N., Matourypour, M., & Ranjbaranet, N. (2017). Therapeutic touch efficacy: A systematic review. *Medical-Surgical Nursing Journal, 5*(4), 52–59.

Classen, C. (2005). Fingerprints. In C. Classen (Ed.), *The book of touch* (pp. 1–9). Berg.

Cohen, L. R. (2011). Time, space and touch at work: Body work and labour process (re)organisation. *Sociology of Health & Illness, 33*(2), 189–205. https://doi.org/10.1111/j.1467-9566.2010.01306.x

Connor, A., & Howett, M. (2009). A conceptual model of intentional comfort touch. *Journal of Holistic Nursing, 27*(2), 127–135.

Coole, D. (2007). Experiencing discourse: Corporeal communicators and the embodiment of power. *The British Journal of Politics and International Relations, 9*(3), 413–433.

Cornell, W. F. (2016). The analyst's body at work: Utilizing touch and sensory experience in psychoanalytic psychotherapies. *Psychoanalytic Perspectives, 13*(2), 168–185. https://doi.org/10.1080/1551806X.2016.1156431

Czarnecka, D. (2020). Instrumental touch: A Foucauldian analysis of women's fitness. *Journal of the Finnish Anthropological Society, 45*(4), 23–43. https://doi.org/10.30676/jfas.v45i4.107794

Davin, L., Thistlethwaite, J., Bartle, E., & Russell, K. (2019). Touch in health professional practice: A review. *The Clinical Teacher, 16*(6), 559–564. https://doi.org/10.1111/tct.13089

Dawson, A., & Dennis, S. (2021). Workplace intimacy. *Anthropology in Action, 28*(1), 1–7.

Dobson, S., Upadhyaya, S., Conyers, I., & Raghavan, R. (2002). Touch in the care of people with profound and complex needs: A review of the literature. *Journal of Intellectual Disabilities, 6*(4), 351–362. https://doi.org/10.1177/1469004702006000402

Douglas, C. (2021). A world of touch in a no-touch pandemic. Living with dementia in a care facility during COVID-19. *Anthropology in Action, 28*(1), 8–15.

Dreyfus, H. L. (2002). 'Intelligence without representation: Merleau-Ponty's critique of mental representation. *Phenomenology and the Cognitive Sciences, 1*, 367–383.

References

Dreyfus, H. L., & Dreyfus, S. E. (1986). *Mind over machine: The power of human intuition and expertise in the era of the computer*. Free Press.

Edwards, S. (1998). An anthropological interpretation of nurses' and patients' per ceptions of the use of space and touch. *Journal of Advanced Nursing, 28*(4), 809–817.

Ennen, E. (2003). Phenomenological coping skills and the striatal memory system. *Phenomenology and the Cognitive Sciences, 2*, 299–325. https://doi.org/10.1023/B:PHEN.0000007368.66888.78

Estabrooks, C. A. (1989). Touch: A nursing strategy in the intensive care unit. *Heart & Lung, 18*(4), 392–401.

Estabrooks, C. A., & Morse, J. M. (1992). Toward a theory of touch: The touching process as acquiring a touching style. *Journal of Advanced Nursing, 17*, 448–456.

Estola, E. (2003). *In the language of the mother: Re-storying the relational moral in teacher's stories*. University of Oulu.

Field, T. (2003). *Touch*. MIT Press.

Fredriksson, L. (1999). Models of relating in a caring conversation: A research synthesis on presence, touch and listening. *Journal of Advanced Nursing, 30*(5), 1167–1176.

Freiberg, A., Girbig, M., Euler, U., Scharfe, J., Nienhaus, A., Freitag, S., & Seidler, A. (2016). Influence of the Kinaesthetics care conception during patient handling on the development of musculoskeletal complaints and diseases – A scoping review. *Journal of Occupational Medicine and Toxicology, 11*(24). https://doi.org/10.1186/s12995-016-0113-x. PMID: 27175210; PMCID: PMC4863326.

Fringer, A., Huth, M., & Hantikainen, V. (2014). Nurses' experiences with the implementation of the Kinaesthetics movement competence training into elderly nursing care: A qualitative focus group study. *Scandinavian Journal of Caring Sciences, 28*(4), 757–766. https://doi.org/10.1111/scs.12108. Epub 2014 Jan 6. PMID: 24387733.

Fuller, B., Simmering, M. J., Marler, L. E., Cox, S. S., Bennett, R. J., & Cheramie, R. A. (2011). Exploring touch as a positive workplace behavior. *Human Relations, 64*(2), 231–256.

Gimlin, D. (2007). What is 'body work'? A review of the literature. *Sociology Compass, 1*, 353–370. https://doi.org/10.1111/j.1751-9020.2007.00015.x

Gleeson, M., & Higgins, A. (2009). Touch in mental health nursing: An exploratory study of nurses' views and perceptions. *Journal of Psychiatric and Mental Health Nursing, 16*(4), 382–389.

Guèguen, N. (2007). Courtship compliance: The effect of touch on women's behavior. *Social Influence, 2*(2), 81–97.

Guindon, M., Packard, R., & Charron, N. (2017). The ethics of touch in the helping relationships. In M. Rovers, J. Malette, & M. Guirguis-Younger (Eds.), *Touch in the helping professions: Research, practice and ethics* (pp. 213–236). University of Ottawa Press. http://www.jstor.org/stable/j.ctv5vdcvd.16

Hassard, J., Holliday, R., & Willmott, H. (Eds.). (2000). *Body and organization*. Sage.

Henneghan, A. M., & Schnyer, R. N. (2015). Biofield therapies for symptom management in palliative and end-of-life care. *American Journal of Hospice and Palliative Medicine, 32*(1), 90–100. https://doi.org/10.1177/1049909113509400

Hertenstein, M. J., Holmes, R., McCullough, M., & Keltner, D. (2009). The communication of emotion via touch. *Emotion, 9*, 566–573.

Hillewaert, S. (2016). Tactics and tactility: A sensory semiotics of handshakes in Central Kenya. *American Anthropologist, 118*(1), 49–66. https://doi.org/10.1111/aman.12517

Hindmarsh, J., & Pilnick, A. (2007). Knowing bodies at work: Embodiment and ephemeral teamwork in Anaesthesia. *Organization Studies, 28*(9), 1395–1416. https://doi.org/10.1177/0170840607068258

Hochschild, A. (1983). *The managed heart*. University of California Press.

Hunter, J., & Struve, M. G. (1998). *The ethical use of touch in psychotherapy*. Sage.

Jakubiak, B. K., & Feeney, B. C. (2017). Affectionate touch to promote relational, psychological, and physical well-being in adulthood: A theoretical model and review of the research. *Personality and Social Psychology Review, 21*(3), 228–252.

Kelly, M. A., Nixon, L., McClurg, C., Scherpbier, A., King, N., & Dornan, T. (2017). Experience of touch in healthcare: A meta-ethnography across the healthcare professions. *Qualitative Health Research*, 1–13. https://doi.org/10.1177/1049732317707726

Keränen, V., Juutinen, J., & Estola, E. (2017). Kosketus päiväkodin kasvattajien kertomuksissa. *Varhaiskasvatuksen Tiedelehti*, 6(2), 249–269.

Kinnunen, T., & Kolehmainen, M. (2019). Touch and affect. Analysing the archive of touch biographies. *Body & Society*, 25(1), 29–56.

Kinnunen, T., & Parviainen, J. (2016). Feeling the right personality. Recruitment consultants' affective decision making in interviews with employee candidates. *Nordic Journal of Working Life Studies*, 6(3), 5–21.

Kinnunen, T., & Seppänen, J. (2009). Oikeaoppinen opettajaruumis. *Naistutkimus*, 4, 6–17.

Klopf, D. W., & McCroskey, J. C. (2007). *Intercultural communication encounters*. Pearson.

Korvajärvi, P. (2016). Ruumiillinen mielihyvä työnä. In J. Parviainen, T. Kinnunen, & I. Kortelainen (Eds.), *Ruumiillisuus ja työelämä. Työruumis jälkiteollisessa taloudessa* (pp. 115–131). Vastapaino.

Lahtinen, R. (2008). *Haptiisit ja hapteemit: Tapaustutkimus kuurosokean henkilön kosketukseen perustuvan kommunikaation kehityksestä*. University of Helsinki.

Leonard, K. E., & Kalman, M. A. (2015). The meaning of touch to patients undergoing chemotherapy. *Oncology Nursing Forum*, 42(5), 517–526.

Leskowitz, E. (2003). Controversies in therapeutic touch. *Seminars in Integrative Medicine*, 1(2), 80–89.

Lindgren, L., Jacobsson, M., & Lämås, K. (2014). Touch massage, a rewarding experience. *Journal of Holistic Nursing*, 32(4), 261–268. https://doi.org/10.1177/0898010114531855

Manning, E. (2007). The politics of touch. In *Sense, movement, sovereignty*. The University of Minneapolis Press.

McCann, K., & McKenna, H. P. (1993). An examination of touch between nurses and elderly patients in a continuing care setting in Northern Ireland. *Journal of Advanced Nursing*, 18(5), 838–846.

Miller, M. J., Franken, N., & Kiefer, K. (2007). Exploring touch communication between coaches and athletes. *Indo-Pacific Journal of Phenomenology*, 7(2), 1–13. https://doi.org/10.1080/20797222.2007.11433953

O'Lynn, C., & Krautscheid, L. (2011). 'How should I touch you?': A qualitative study of attitudes on intimate touch in nursing care. *The American Journal of Nursing*, 111(3), 24–33. https://doi.org/10.1097/10.1097/01.NAJ.0000395237.83851.79. PMID: 21346463.

Papathanassoglou, E. D. E., & Mpouzika, M. D. A. (2012). Interpersonal touch: Physiological effects in critical care. *Biological Research for Nursing*, 14(4), 431–443.

Paterson, M. (2004). Caresses, excesses, intimacies and estrangements. *Journal of the Theoretical Humanities*, 9(1), 165–177. https://doi.org/10.1080/0969725042000232478

Pink, S., Morgan, J., & Dainty, A. (2014). The safe hand: Gels, water, gloves and the materiality of tactile knowing. *Journal of Material Culture*, 19(4), 425–442. https://doi.org/10.1177/1359183514555053

Routasalo, P. (1997). *Touch in the nursing care of elderly patients*. University of Turku.

Routasalo, P. (1999). Physical touch in nursing studies: A literature review. *Journal of Advanced Nursing*, 30(4), 843–850.

Royeen, C. R., & Mu, K. (2003). Stability of tactile defensiveness across cultures: European and American children's responses to the touch inventory for elementary school aged children. *Occupational Therapy International*, 10(3), 165–174. https://doi.org/10.1002/oti.183. PMID: 12900789.

Sandnes, L., & Uhrenfeldt, L. (2022). Caring touch in intensive care nursing: A qualitative study. *International Journal of Qualitative Studies on Health and Well-Being*, 17(1), 1–11. https://doi.org/10.1080/17482631.2022.2092964

Schlage, B. (2021). Touch and affect regulation. Postural integration, trauma skills, and tools for body-oriented psychotherapy. *International Body Psychotherapy Journal. The Art and Science of Somatic Praxis*, 20(1), 50–60.

Schneider, E. F., & Patterson, P. P. (2010). You've got that magic touch: Integrating the sense of touch into early childhood services. *Young Exceptional Children*, 13(5), 17–27. https://doi.org/10.1177/1096250610384706

Straughan, E. R. (2012). Facing touch in the beauty salon: Corporeal anxiety. In M. Paterson & M. Dodge (Eds.), *Touching space, placing touch* (pp. 89–101). Routledge.
Styrman, T., & Torniainen, M. (2018). *Kunnioittavan kosketuksen käsikirja. Ammatillinen hoitokohtaaminen sosiaali- ja terveysalalla*. PS-kustannus.
Sutton, J., McIlwain, D., Christensen, W., & Geeves, A. (2011). Applying intelligence to the reflexes: Embodied skills and habits between Dreyfus and Descartes. *Journal of the British Society for Phenomenology, 42*(1), 78–103. https://doi.org/10.1080/00071773.2011.11006732
Suvilehto, J. T., Nummenmaa, L., Harada, T., Dunbar, R. I. M., Hari, R., Turner, R., Sadato, N., & Kitada, R. (2019). Cross-cultural similarity in relationship-specific social touching. *Proceedings of the Royal Society B, 286*, 20190467. https://doi.org/10.1098/rspb.2019.0467
Tanner, L. (2017). *Embracing touch in dementia care: A person-centred approach to touch and relationships*. Jessica Kingsley Publishers.
Van Dongen, E., & Elema, R. (2001). The art of touching: The culture of "body work" in nursing. *Anthropology & Medicine, 8*(2–3), 149–161.
Vortherms, R. C. (1991). Clinically improving communication through touch. *Journal of Gerontological Nursing, 17*(5), 6–10.
Wolf, Z. R., Bailey, D. N., & Stubin, C. A. (2022). Bodywork and nursing practice: Development of a bodywork in nursing practice instrument. *Nursing Forum, 57*, 509–529. https://doi.org/10.1111/nuf.12703
Wolkowitz, C. (2006). *Bodies at work*. SAGE.
Yon, Y., Mikton, C. R., Gassoumis, Z. D., & Wilber, K. H. (2017). Elder abuse prevalence in community settings: A systematic review and meta-analysis. *The Lancet Global Health, 5*, e147–e156.

Further Reading

Brandstetter, G., Egert, G., & Zubarik, S. (2013). *Touching and being touched: Kinesthesia and empathy in dance and movement*. Walter de Gruyter.
Green, B., & Hopwood, N. (Eds.). (2015). *The body in professional practice, learning and education*. Springer.
Field, T. (2003). *Touch*. MIT Press.
Fulkerson, M. (2014). *The first sense: A philosophical study of the sense of touch*. MIT Press.
Hertenstein, M. J., & Weiss, S. J. (Eds.). (2011). *The handbook of touch: Neuroscience, behavioral, and health perspectives*. Springer Publishing Company.
Montagu, A. (1971). *Touching*. Columbia University Press.
Walters, S. (2014). *Rhetorical touch: Disability, identification, haptics*. University of South Carolina Press.

Socialisation into Touch Cultures

Abstract

This chapter introduces socialisation processes through which we adopt touch practices. We address primary socialisation during early childhood and secondary socialisation as cultural learning about norms of touch. We discuss primary attachment styles and affective repertoires, which in turn reproduce certain touch patterns in later life. Attachment styles and affective repertoires also impact on the ways in which people encounter one another through touch in their roles as clients and professionals. We recall that touch practices develop in historical, ideological, economic, material and social conditions that comprise comprehensive 'skinscapes'. We argue that tactile encounters in client work cannot be understood or even performed unless one considers these factors that are present in encounters. We consider cultural differences regarding manners of touch, gendered touch practices and conceptions of proper physical proximity. It is important to understand cultural variations if we wish to develop equal, humane and culturally sensitive client work practices.

Introduction

This chapter introduces various dimensions of the socialisation processes through which we adopt particular touch practices. We address primary socialisation during early childhood and secondary socialisation as cultural learning about norms of touch. We first discuss how touch habits are transferred across families and generations through childcare practices. These practices produce different primary attachment styles and affective repertoires, which in turn reproduce certain touch patterns in later life. Learnt attachment styles and affective repertoires also impact on the ways in which people encounter one another through touch in their roles as clients and professionals.

We recall that touch practices develop in historical, ideological, economic, material and social conditions that comprise comprehensive 'skinscapes'. Professional touch practices, as part of a general touch culture, are patterned by these circumstances. Therefore, tactile encounters in client work cannot be understood or even performed unless one considers the cultural factors that are always present in encounters. We consider cultural differences regarding manners of touch, gendered touch practices, and conceptions of proper physical proximity. It is important to consider these cultural variations—including differences with regard to ethnicity, gender, age, class, sexuality and emotional capital gained during childhood—if we wish to develop equal, humane and culturally sensitive client work practices.

Learning Objectives
This chapter is intended to help you identify the meaning of cultural learning for touch practices and appraise its effects on client encounters. After reading this chapter, you should be able to:

- discuss how human senses are culturally and historically constructed and in what kind of 'skinscape' we live.
- indicate the importance of primary and secondary socialisation to manners, meanings and experiences of touch.
- explain how touch is culturally gendered and sexualised and how it may affect professional touch practices.
- estimate how to respect cultural differences while still finding ways to overcome seeming barriers.

3.1 Primary Socialisation into Touch

Touch is the earliest sensory modality to develop in the human body, and it functions as a basis for the perception of one's own body and relational self. Experiences of touch during early childhood have far-reaching consequences for tactile relations in later life and become obvious in professional contexts too (Davis et al., 2017). A baby is concretely taken into the world among others through touch. Touch is critical for the infant's survival and bonding during the newborn period, and it continues to be the primary channel of communication for about the first two years. The basis of one's 'attachment style' and related touch habits lies in childhood experiences when parents and other caregivers respond to an infant's needs with different gestures. Feeding, putting to sleep, nappy-changing, bathing, dressing, playing and other caring practices are necessary parts of daily childcare, all performed by touching. Most babies seek attention by crying, and caregivers ideally respond to this by picking the baby up and holding, caressing, kissing, carrying and rocking it. 'Attachment behaviours' such as crying are adaptive responses to separation from the primary 'attachment figure' and perhaps also from other caregivers that guarantee the survival of the baby, which is wholly dependent upon the care and protection of adults.

3.1 Primary Socialisation into Touch

The early tactile (and other sensory) responses of the attachment figure (caregiver) mould the ways in which the baby seeks to gain their attention and help. The baby also learns what kind of response to expect from the caregiver(s) and how to comfort itself while separated from them. The behaviour of primary attachment figures (usually the parents) and secondary caregivers (e.g. healthcare and education professionals) significantly contributes to how the child perceives itself and also to its subsequent close relationships during adulthood. The attachment style manifests itself through the ways in which the child desires to be in physical and emotional proximity to the attachment figure and the kind of anxiety that occurs in the absence of that attachment figure. The attachment style is also reflected in the ways the attachment figure serves as a secure base for the child in the face of fear or threat and while the child is exploring the surrounding environment (Cherry, 2022).

Originally developed by the British psychoanalyst John Bowlby (e.g. 1988), attachment theory distinguishes between two basic attachment styles: *secure* and *insecure*. The secure attachment style develops when the caregiver reacts to the baby quickly and responds to its need for physical and emotional proximity and care. Securely attached babies become upset when separated from caregivers and are happy again when the caregivers return. In a secure attachment, the baby learns it can rely on the attentiveness and availability of the caregiver, and consequently it mostly feels secure and confident. This confidence is reflected in its social behaviour, so a securely attached baby is likely to explore the environment, engage with other people and enjoy play with other children. After childhood, a securely attached person tends to trust others and communicate with them easily, without experiencing feelings of inferiority, while remaining able to self-reflect. In an intimate relationship, they can seek and offer emotional support.

The insecure attachment style, on the other hand, develops when the baby learns that the caregiver is not available when needed and/or responds to the baby's needs in ambivalent or harmful ways. There are three main insecure attachment styles, although their terms vary to some extent. The first is the *avoidant* (or 'dismissive-avoidant' or 'anxious-avoidant') insecure attachment style, which the baby adopts if the caregiver is rarely or never available when needed. A strict, emotionally distant or absent caregiver will lead the baby to believe that it is not worth noticing and caring for, and that the attachment figure's attention can only be gained (if at all) through withdrawing behaviour rather than by reaching out. When separated from the attachment figure, the baby does not seem to react with strong feelings either to their absence or to their return. In adulthood, an avoidantly attached person often has difficulties sharing their thoughts, feelings and physical intimacy with partners. In general, they may avoid investing in social and romantic relationships, instead having a strong sense of independence and mistrust. However, avoidantly attached persons may also be tolerant and open-minded with regard to sexual issues.

The second insecure attachment style is *ambivalent* (or 'anxious-ambivalent' or 'anxious-preoccupied'), which develops because of inconsistency in the caregiver's responses to the baby's expressed needs. The caregiver may alternate between being overly coddling and being detached or indifferent, so the baby cannot be sure what to expect. If separated from the attachment figure, the baby displays considerable distress and is not comforted by the caregiver's return. In adulthood, ambivalently attached persons often feel reluctant to form intimate relationships and become extremely stressed by relationship break-ups. They tend to be jealous and distrustful due to poor self-esteem.

The third type of insecure attachment style is *disorganised* (or 'anxious-disorganised'), which the baby adopts if the relationship with the attachment figure(s) is extremely ambivalent. The disorganised attachment style is usually related to trauma caused by serious neglect or abuse that leads the child to fear the caregiver(s). The baby or child displays avoidance, resistance, confusion and apprehension in the presence of the caregiver. This confusion and unpredictable behaviour often continue in adult intimate partnerships, because the disorganised attachment style gives rise to tendencies to be aloof and independent, and at the same time clingy and emotional (Mandriota, 2021).

Attachment styles are internal working models that tend to serve as learnt patterns for intimate and other close relationships. They can be considered from the point of view of touch because, as stated earlier, touch practices result in and from specific attachment styles—although we must bear in mind that attachment and touch are not synonymous. Attachment theory has developed in a Western cultural context—where it represents specifically middle-class morality regarding 'good' and 'bad' gendered parenthood (Keller, 2018)—but its main idea is applicable cross-culturally to a certain extent. Anthropologists have long been interested in how different childcare and child-rearing practices—which are notably performed through touch—and related value and belief systems produce personalities that are in accordance with cultural ideals regarding gender and social class, for example (see Box 3.1).

> **Box 3.1 Culture and Personality**
> In her celebrated study of New Guinea, Margaret Mead (1935) compared childcare practices and adult temperaments in three societies: Arapesh, Mundugumor and Tchambuli. She argued that Arapesh society displayed both extremely gentle constant touching of children and non-aggressivity among adults, whereas Mundugumor society displayed harsh and distancing childcare practices and aggressive, warring adults. These observations opened a path to understanding how sociocultural factors modify selfhood and personhood. Ruth Benedict (1934), one of the founders of psychological anthropology, stated in her 'culture and personality' theory that all cultures favour certain personality traits that are compatible with their core cultural values and aesthetics, which comprise identifiable cultural patterns of thought and action. She drew a distinction between 'rational Apollonian' and 'hedonist Dionysian' cultures, for example.
>
> Although both Mead and Benedict have been criticised for generalising too easily, numerous studies have addressed the connection between touching practices and personality traits in adulthood, including psychical and physiological disorders.

From an anthropological perspective, it is not justifiable to draw a distinction between touch culture in the abstract and individual experiences of touch or observable touch practices. Nevertheless, culture cannot be reduced to individual experiences and behaviours or vice versa. Rather, culture consists of lived individual variables. Experiences and practices of touch (re)constitute cultures all the time, as Taina Kinnunen and Marjo Kolehmainen (2019, pp. 3, 6) state: 'Culture does not straightforwardly regulate touch; touch also constitutes bodies and their affective interconnectedness', and 'culture does not provide us with a mere collection of norms, but rather foregrounds affective relations where we experience touch in embodied and psychical ways'. Thus, one's experiences of and responses to touch depend on one's socialisation into touch and specific situations of touch which reconstitute culture. The cultural patterns and situational factors that contribute to touch practices are not static because changing ideological, social, political, economic and material factors resonate in them. In one historical era, for example, ideologies and institutional policies may favour punishing or controlling touch in childcare or care for the disabled, whereas in another era those practices may be sanctioned.

One way of making sense of how attachment styles work in real life in cultural and historical contexts is to scrutinise people's lifelong experiences of touch. We did this in our study of Finnish touch culture, which was based on touch biographies—life stories narrated from the angle of touch experiences. Our analysis of touch biographies revealed that people have different 'affective repertoires' that are enacted in, through and in retreat from touch throughout their life course (Kinnunen & Kolehmainen, 2019). Although individual touch experiences and the related affective repertoires presumably vary across cultures, the results of three distinct affective repertoires are worth considering in any cultural context.

First, some people associate touch with warmth and care because their experiences of touch have predominantly been loving and pleasant. Touch is a positive life resource for them, and they experience it as a natural way of expressing and receiving affection. These narratives speak to secure attachment styles and relational wellbeing—a kind of 'emotional capital, i.e. reservoirs of positive, shared experiences' (Jakubiak & Feeney, 2017, p. 7) that helps to create affectionate relationships and to endure and resolve difficulties in them. Second, there are persons for whom touch has predominantly meant pain and humiliation during their life course. Consequently, their affective repertoire is by no means an empowering reservoir: touch has drained them. Among our older research participants, physical punishment had been a relatively common experience because early twentieth-century childcare doctrines had encouraged it. However, many young women in their twenties had also experienced harsh violence from parents and/or intimate partners, and school bullying was also widely reported in the biographies. In some cases, these affective repertoires seemed to refer to insecure attachment styles, probably of the ambivalent or disorganised varieties. However, it must be noted that a child that is securely attached to its caregivers may also face violence during adulthood—the culture may provide other impulses towards violent behaviour.

The third type of affective repertoire can best be described in terms of lack. The absence of caring touch had afflicted several of our participants during some or all of their lives. Many referred to this lack as a 'haunting' experience that had confused them and caused them pain, often without their being able to name it. These affective repertoires suggest avoidant attachment styles, which some commentators have argued are more common in Finland than in other countries (Tirkkonen, 2015). This can be explained by events in Finland's twentieth-century history, including exceptionally difficult wartime experiences and a period of famine. Combined with a reliance on authoritarian paediatric doctrines, these events led to a communal failure to provide sufficient care and security. Survival was a matter of hard work and willpower, and the social virtue of 'coping alone' developed as a survival strategy. Although the welfare state has now made Finland a very different country, a residue of this affective history is still being transmitted across the generations, as our participants' touch biographies revealed. This Finnish case study exemplifies how attachment styles are produced by touching practices and their affective matterings in specific social, cultural and material contexts.

Individuals seldom have a clear or categorical attachment style, and their experiences of touch are usually multiple. However, individual affective repertoires do vary and are also a source of social inequality. Protective touch experienced during childhood is the foundation for respect for one's own bodily territory and the creation of trusting relationships. A neglected or abused child may not recognise its boundaries and may therefore become prone to exploitation in later life. Individual experiences of touch may also significantly impact on how a person as a patient or client is willing and able to receive any kind of touch from professionals. We argue that attachment theory and the theory of culture-bound affective repertoires offer a conceptual framework that can illuminate how a client's past experiences with caregivers and others might influence transactions between the client and a professional (see Meyer & Pilkonis, 2001).

Luke Tanner (2017) has observed that different attachment styles can show up in the ways in which people with dementia experience therapeutic massage. Indeed, his observations may perhaps be extended to all contexts of professional touch. He emphasises that it is important for a professional to be aware of different attachment styles and recognise the behaviours related to them. This enables the professional to recognise the client's attachment style and thus to apply their touch in the manner that will benefit the client most. Tanner states that avoidantly attached persons usually benefit more from indirect touch than from intentional touching in close physical proximity. The occasional touching involved in shared activities, touch via objects or massage are often more suitable than hugging, holding hands or sitting side by side.

People with ambivalent or disorganised attachment styles, on the other hand, may express their needs in inconsistent and controversial ways that often confuse others. A client may be clingy, consistently seeking closeness and soothing touch from the professional, and at the next moment they may respond dismissively, anxiously or aggressively to the same professional touch. It has been acknowledged that recognising the client's attachment style also plays a key role in psychiatric counselling for individuals and couples. Isaac Davis and colleagues (2017) stress the special needs of insecurely attached clients, with whom certain touch therapies, self-touch methods and canine-assisted touch can be utilised successfully. On the other hand, it has also been proposed that any kind of physical contact is risky in psychiatric counselling for 'those with poor attachment histories' (Harrison et al., 2012, p. 278).

An awareness of attachment theory makes it easier for the professional to understand their own touch style at work (Sect. 2.4) and to process their own affects during professional encounters. Although a skilful professional can partly control their own affective responses to touch and use touch in multiple ways while respecting the principle of equality, their socialisation and experiences of touch will inevitably influence their professional self. Due to personal experiences, affective repertoires of touch vary among professionals too. The teachers and nurses we interviewed seemed to be very conscious of their own styles and repertoires as both private and professional persons, which they often considered to be related. Some described themselves as 'touch people', while others considered themselves to be reserved touchers. Jonna was one of those nurses who assessed herself as a touch person.

> After all, not every nurse wants to touch, but it's a must when you read the instructions 'put skin cream on the client's feet'. But on the other hand, it's natural for me, even if there are no instructions, that you should put skin cream on the client's feet, so I might moisturise their feet in any case. (Jonna, Finnish nurse)

'Eini', instead, thought that she was not a touch person. She had retired from her work as a nurse and reflected impressively on her professional and private touching selves in her touch biography. She began her story by saying that she had become used to touching her patients 'technically' and was even able to provide a 'tender and encouraging' touch for some of them. But, Eini wrote, she touched her children, husband, father or friends not because she wanted to, but 'because of them'. She explained her experiences of touch during adulthood in terms of the affective atmosphere in which she had grown up as a child. Her parents and grandparents had been 'emotionally cold'. Her parents had separated, sent the children to foster homes, then got back together and brought some of the children back home. Eini related that there was 'always a contentious and threatening atmosphere' at home, and that her parents had never taken her into their laps or even been happy about her. She also believed she had been sexually abused: although she could not remember the events, she presumed the strong anxiety that had emerged during psychotherapy as an adult signalled a traumatic experience. Eini said she had always found it natural to touch animals and that she could feel tenderness towards them, unlike children. She reported she had had only two 'unconditionally gentle and caring touches' during her whole lifetime: one from a male doctor during her childhood and one from a physiotherapist as an adult:

> This seemingly safe and gentle old man rubbed my neck with his big hands, the neck recovered immediately, and I wished that the man would stay to live with us. It is my first memory of a good touch – a physiotherapist folded me in her accepting, warm embrace. In one group situation, I was deeply moved and was crying uncontrollably. This gentle woman

kept me in her lap on the floor and I could cry until I felt better. Such unconditional caring I had never experienced before. (Eini, Finnish nurse)

This case exemplifies not only the correspondence a professional can perceive between their private and professional selves, but also how the touch of a professional in client work can dramatically widen an individual's affective repertoire of touch. This kind of 'affective peak' in experiences of healing touch can sometimes even slightly reshape an individual's attachment style, if they become conscious of that attachment style and have an idea of the direction in which to develop it. This can also have consequences for one's professional identity or change one's professional touch style per se, as some of our interviewees emphasised. Sari, the nurse who had worked for a long time in home care, described how she had gradually widened her own tactile and affective repertoires through conscious self-reflection and relearning. Sari had been raised by parents who seldom touched her warmly, and she had realised that her personal history had affected her professional identity and touching style. In her private life, Sari still did not feel like a 'hugger'. However, she had started to diversify the intentions behind her professional touch from instrumental to connecting and caring touch (see Sect. 2.1), because she had noticed that some of her elderly clients clearly need those kinds of touch. Sari had also learned to identify clients who did not want to be touched unless there was an obvious reason:

> I'm not that kind of person at all who goes and gives hugs, I don't have that kind of habit like some of my friends, for example, have – I find it very embarrassing if somebody comes and hugs me, I haven't been taught that – I have tried to add it in my work – because you see it clearly that elderly and older persons, who are so lonely, need touching – And when you get to know these clients when there are long care relationships, so you get to realise who likes it when you go and say hello or goodbye by touching their shoulder.
>
> You work through your personality anyway. It is for the sake of your professional role that you touch, because you work in physical proximity. You basically touch during every visit when you give them their morning bath, change their incontinence pants, spread lotion on their skin, so it must feel natural to some extent, you wouldn't choose this profession otherwise. But whether you also give something extra from yourself, that's every one's own decision. (Sari, Finnish nurse)

3.2 Culture-Bound Touch

> Do we learn a 'mother touch' along with a mother tongue? A tactile code of communication that underpins the ways we engage with other people and the world? No doubt we do. Our hands and bodies learn to 'speak' a certain language of touch, a language shaped by culture and inflected by individuals. We learn what to touch, how to touch, and what significance to give different kinds of touch. Laden with meaning and bound by rules, touch has what could be called a vocabulary and a grammar. (Classen, 2005, p. 13)

A newborn baby is literally attached to its parents and other people through touch in a particular place and time. The baby immediately starts a lifelong socialisation process as it imitates, absorbs and improvises touching etiquettes. Its attachment to its caregivers and its socialisation into the nurturing family through touch are embedded with cultural and historical meanings. Touch is a historically and culturally structured sense, sensation and act, and it is not performed or experienced in universally congruent ways. The above-cited Canadian author, Constance Classen, who edited *The book of touch* (Classen, 2005), crystallises this in the idea of the 'mother touch' that we learn as members of society. The consequence of a failure to internalise the tactile regime is that others will not only reject you as alien but will feel seriously offended by you (Cranny-Francis, 2011, p. 468). Socialisation happens largely subconsciously; we usually only become aware of the cultural norms of touch when somebody breaks the rules—for example, in an intercultural encounter. A northern European or North American might feel confused on meeting an Italian who greeted them by kissing their cheeks and then kept touching their hand, shoulder or leg every now and again while they chatted. Even within cultures, individuals of different generations, social classes and religions may follow different tactile regimes, not to mention different touch norms across genders.

By the term 'culture' we mean the set of conceptions, meanings and practices that people adopt through learning and share in their social, historical and spatial context. Cultures exist in geographically confined areas but cannot be reduced to them: they exist in multisited, dispersed locations and are renewed through physical and mediated communication (Gupta & Ferguson, 1992). In everyday thinking, culture is usually associated with ethnicity, whereby individual and social identities overlap but are not synonymous. The term 'culture' can refer to the collection of beliefs and practices of any social group whose members share those beliefs and practices and produce and feel togetherness through them. All people are socialised into some kind of *body culture*: socially shared ways of understanding, conceptualising, treating, presenting and valuing the body in relation to other human and non-human bodies (Burton, 2001). As the French anthropologist Marcel Mauss (1936/1973) stated almost a hundred years ago, all people are also socialised into certain cultural 'body techniques': ways to use and move the body in everyday life.

Variations in body techniques in different natural and societal environments mean that people 'inhabit different sensory worlds', as Edward T. Hall (1963) proposed in his celebrated study of 'proxemics'. Hall used this term to refer to the ways in which people spatially regulate and experience communication 'zones'. He distinguished four zones of proxemics: intimate, personal, social and public. The intimate zone (15–45 cm) is normally reserved for sexual partners and family members. In this 'kissing zone', bodily aroma and body heat can be sensed. In the personal zone (46–130 cm), it is possible to maintain focused eye contact and to touch the body parts that are usually perceived as socially acceptable: hands, arms and shoulders. The social zone (130–350 cm), sometimes called the 'proper work relation zone', enables eye and voice contact but not tactile contact. The public zone is the most remote communication zone, where interaction happens mainly through the auditory and visual senses.

As this book deals with touch as a working tool, we will naturally focus our discussion on the first two zones: the intimate and personal zones. When discussing multisensory communication, such as the use of movement, voice and sight in the context of touch, we will also briefly mention the social and public zones. In healthcare and early childhood education and care contexts, contact zones have been discussed in terms of the boundaries that define 'safe spaces' and 'territories', which should be respected when one is 'invading' the patient's or child's personal or intimate zone. Contrary to everyday norms, in healthcare and early childhood education contexts, we have exceptional permission to invade a stranger's intimate zone and touch even the most intimate body parts (e.g. Estabrooks & Morse, 1992). Besides formal training, this permission is based on the governance of the profession and the internal norms and practices of each working organisation, which vary across countries and cultures. Indeed, Hall and many other researchers have noted that contact zones and non-verbal bodily communications, especially touch behaviours, vary across and within cultures. Several reasons have been proposed for this variation: climate and related biological processes and changes in the human body; traditional values of collectivism or individualism; power relations and roles between genders, religions and political systems (Andersen, 2011; Dibiase & Gunnoe, 2004). Obviously, many of these factors (and others) influence touch cultures.

Researchers usually divide cultures, cultural areas or ethnic groups into contact and non-contact cultures. Contact cultures include Mediterranean countries, southern and eastern Europe, most Arab and Islamic groups, Russian people, most Jewish societies, Central and Latin Americans, and several African societies. Northern Europe, North America, Japan, China, South Korea and some other East and South-East Asian societies are categorised as non-contact cultures. Some studies have suggested that in the United States, black people seem to use tactile contact in more complex ways in greetings, for example, compared with white people. Although there is no comprehensive cross-cultural comparative research, a fair number of empirical studies have indicated differences between contact and non-contact cultures. From observations of same-gender and cross-gender touching behaviour between and among adults and children in public spaces such as cafeterias and parks, for example, it has been confirmed that French, Italian, Puerto Rican, Cuban and Costa Rican people touch each other during conversation much more than do English, German or North American people (Argyle, 1988; Field, 2003; Gallace & Spence, 2010; Klopf & McCroskey, 2007; Manusov, 2017).

Another way of dividing touch cultures into two major categories is 'low-touch' collectivist versus 'high-touch' individualistic cultures. Mexican culture and Asian cultures found in Japan, Singapore, Taiwan and Hong Kong and are often perceived as typical collectivist cultures, where the 'we' identity is much more important than 'I' identity. In these cultures, open touching in public spaces is easily interpreted as intrusive, selfish and immature, unlike in individualistic cultures, where the same tactile manners are usually associated with warmth, care and affiliation (Andersen, 2011). However, it is noteworthy that individualist cultures encompass quite different touch cultures—for example, contact-intensive southern European countries and non-contact Scandinavian countries—so this dichotomy is rough and somewhat controversial. It should also be remembered that certain occasions, such as spiritual rituals, games, sports, feasts, accidents or outbreaks of disease, are examples of situations where different norms of touch may apply compared with everyday life. In many cultures and societies, touch habits also vary between rural and urban communities, older and younger generations, upper and lower social classes, and different ethnic, religious and language groups.

There may be totally divergent norms of cross-gender touch in public compared with same-gender touch. In Arab cultures, same-gender bodily contact is understood as a sign of friendship rather than as sexually loaded. Kissing, hand-holding and embracing between men are common sights everywhere, whereas one rarely sees cross-gender touching (in many countries, women are less visible in public spaces in any case). In Anglo-Saxon cultures, by contrast, it is almost impossible to see men touching each other in public, except during sports or in exceptionally emotional situations of happiness or grief. On the other hand, cross-gender touching is commonly accepted, and touch between females is more acceptable than between males. In one study, researchers observed 103 greetings in American airports. They found that all the encounters in which a female person was involved included a kiss or an embrace, while men usually either shook hands or did not touch at all (Greenbaum & Rosenfeld, 1980; see also Dolinski, 2010).

It is probable that gendered touch norms vary across social classes and generations in all societies. For example, some decades ago the performance of 'real' working-class manhood in rural Finland meant that a father would avoid caressing or kissing his own child in public. The differences in touch norms between genders became evident for 'Markku', a transman whose blog post described the transformation his touch habits underwent when his gender was corrected:

> You had to leave a polite distance with boys. You had to realise the change of your status and that some people got confused if you hugged them the same way as before. So: the touch zone must be kept as minimal as possible when hugging. The shoulders can touch each other, and the arms can touch the back. You have to keep your chest detached from the other person's chest, legs as far as possible, and keep your pelvis back. No stroking, patting the back is allowed, even favoured. Hugs must be kept brief. (Finnish man, quoted in Kinnunen, 2013)

The above-cited example demonstrates how culturally 'valid' genders and classes are *done* by touch practices. In this sense, it can be argued that gender is 'performative': a series of repeated embodied performances that include regulated touch behaviours. It must be noted that gender performances change over time; they are reproduced. Throughout Europe in the Middle Ages, kissing, embracing and holding hands were common tokens of goodwill between all genders and ages. In the United States, a hundred years ago, male affection was shown by touch much more than is the case today, including by holding hands, bathing or sleeping together (Bourke, 2009). During the twentieth century, behaviour changed when homosexuality became categorised as a sexual identity—a pathological one. The paradox now is that homosexuality is illegal in many Arab countries, whereas the pathological label barely exists in the Anglo-Saxon world today.

The case of Japan also demonstrates how difficult it can be for a Westerner to understand the nuanced meanings of an unfamiliar touch culture. In Japan, adults rarely intentionally touch each other in public, but in crowded spaces such as buses, trains and stations, they can remain comfortable in close physical contact, sometimes even leaning on each other while taking a nap. This perhaps stems from the specific meanings of co-sleeping (*soine*) in Japanese culture, which comprise different co-sleeping patterns ranging from the family bed—Japanese children up to the age of 15 years often sleep between their parents—to business trips. In kindergartens, it is a professional practice to co-sleep with children in order to provide them with a 'family-like *skinship*' because children are believed to need physical proximity to adults, as one headteacher told Diana Adis Tahhan (2008) during an ethnographic interview. Researchers often point out that Japanese parents, especially mothers, generally maintain close tactile contact with their children throughout their childhood (e.g. Field, 2003).

The religious core of Japanese thinking is Shinto, in which body and mind are not separated but understood as a sacred whole. Touch is not sexualised in the Western sense, and it is therefore not tabooed in client work. Skin is more open than closed, and bodily boundaries are fluid and extend into space. Physical closeness and touch are seen as natural ways of feeling the 'mutual vibration' in a shared space, although affectionate touch between intimate partners is much more controlled than in Western cultures (Sakiyama & Koch, 2003; Tahhan, 2008). On the other hand, it has been observed that Japanese people—like Finns—touch each other quite freely when they are drunk, but not when they are sober. In both cultures, mixed bathing and saunas (usually while naked) lack the sexual implications found in many other cultures. The bathwater or hot steam spreads among the bodies and provides a collective bodily sense, even a feeling of sacred togetherness with the other bathers, the water and (as is often the case in Finnish summer cottages) the natural environment that surrounds the sauna.

Cultural conceptions regarding whom it is acceptable, pleasant or unpleasant to touch extend beyond gender. Strict touch prohibitions concern the royal family in the UK as well as the lowest caste in India, albeit for the opposite reasons. In the former case, the prohibition on touch expresses honour and respect for the highest class in the social hierarchy; in the latter, the avoidance of touch expresses a dissociation from the 'impure' Dalits (formerly known as Untouchables), which strengthened during the COVID-19 pandemic (see Satyogi, 2021). In many societies people may avoid touching the severely ill, alcoholics, drug addicts or criminals without necessarily even realising they are doing so, and this inevitably marks and reproduces status in the social hierarchy. In today's Western society, where youth is idealised, the body of an elderly person may be categorised as repellent, even terrifying, and difficult to touch. The ageing body is associated with decay, illness and death, and its wrinkles and leakages are associated with dirt (Isaksen, 2002). Ageing has become an 'illness' that requires medical interventions such as plastic surgery to prevent its horrifying processes (Kinnunen, 2010). Discourses surrounding young and ageing bodies contain socially shared conceptions and beliefs about what kinds of bodies are easy and desirable to touch and what affective responses they 'deserve', such as attraction or disgust (cf. Ahmed, 2004). Therefore, regardless of whether the person we touch is known to us, our own bodies do not respond to touches with all other bodies in the same way. The affects that are actualised in tactile contact are informed by cultural discourses regarding different bodies, such as verbal and visual representations of ages, genders, classes, sizes, ethnicities, skin colours, sexualities and styles (cf. Kyrölä, 2014).

The social is embedded in our psychophysiological responses to touch in professional contexts too, even if we seldom realise it. One marker of cultural discourses regarding 'touchable' and 'untouchable' bodies can be recognised in nurse education, for example. The nursing teachers we interviewed told us that few students were interested in specialising in elderly care at the outset of their studies (see also Field, 2003, p. 29). Fortunately, a practical training period in elderly care could persuade them to change their minds. Of course, there are also students whose explicit aim right at the start of their studies is to become geriatric nurses, and some of our student interviewees fell into this category. In their practical training, they had noticed that some students and workers in geriatric care were only willing to touch older adults while wearing gloves. The interviewees would be in tears while they told us about this: how could something that felt so important, natural and easy for them be unnatural and repulsive to someone else?

In the internal hierarchy of hospital nursing, touch-intensive work on wards for elderly patients may be less valued than work on other wards. In the context of psychiatric hospital nursing, work on wards for elderly patients may be perceived as 'too quiet and easy' and 'not real psychiatry' compared with psychiatric emergency care. Hospital geriatric nursing is a position from which a nurse is expected to move on into something more prestigious (e.g. Van Dongen & Riekje, 2001). Another embodiment of cultural beliefs concerning the professional touch of ageing bodies was found in a study that explored non-verbal communication between hospitalised older adults and hospital staff in Cameroon. Esther L. Wanko Keutchafo and colleagues (2022) noted that some nurses avoided physical proximity or tactile contact with end-of-life patients because of the fear of becoming a target of witchcraft performed by the dying.

Only a few comparative studies, with limited empirical evidence, have systematically examined the influence of cultural differences regarding touch behaviour on cross-cultural professional-client relations. However, cultural, religious and ethnic backgrounds need to be taken into account as far as possible in professional encounters with clients and their family members, to prevent misunderstandings. The term 'multicultural' itself contains the idea of sensitivity to difference, and nowadays *cultural sensitivity* is included in many countries' legal-ethical principles regarding healthcare, social work and education practices. Cultural diversity or difference is ideally respected as a standard in the teaching of communication skills to professionals, rather than being treated as an adjustment to existing practices. Building awareness of and sensitivity to cultural differences is vitally important if we wish to develop *cultural competence*. According to Stella Williams and colleagues (2013, p. 43), cultural competence refers to 'Culturally and Linguistically Appropriate Services', defined by the US Department of Health and Human Services as 'a set of congruent behaviours, attitudes, and policies that come together in a system, agency, or among professionals that enable effective work in cross-cultural situations'. This comes close to the conceptual and practical guidelines issued by the Finnish Institute for Health and Welfare for work in multicultural environments (Box 3.2).

> **Box 3.2 Cultural Sensitivity (Slightly Modified from the Guidelines by the Finnish Institute for Health and Welfare, 2021)**
>
> The concept of cultural competence refers to respect for people of any cultural background, and the creation and fostering of an atmosphere of non-discrimination in society. It also means the provision, availability and accessibility of services in a manner that takes account of the varying needs of people of different backgrounds.
>
> The cultural competence of professionals comprises cultural awareness, knowledge, skills, encounters and motivation, which involves reflecting one's own cultural habits and values with the habits and values of other cultures.
>
> Cultural sensitivity is also related to cultural competence. Cultural sensitivity refers to professionals' culturally respectful interpersonal skills, and respectful verbal and non-verbal encounters and communications between professionals and clients in a manner that respects the right of each party to express their culture, be accepted and be heard.
>
> Thus, cultural sensitivity refers to the willingness, ability and sensitivity required to understand people of different backgrounds. Culturally sensitive services do not entail the provision of separate services for each target group; instead, it means making services flexible to meet the needs of diverse clients.
>
> Although cultural competence and cultural sensitivity are often linked to the work of social and healthcare professionals, all forms of customer work should take them into account.
>
> The premises of cultural sensitivity in client work are:
>
> - perceiving one's own cultural background, conceptions and manners and using this as the basis for increasing one's understanding of other cultures;
> - respecting diversity;
> - taking an interest in different cultures;
> - reflecting on the effects and significance of one's cultural background for oneself and one's personal attitudes;
> - finding the courage to encounter clients as individuals rather than as representatives of certain cultures;
> - being open and patient;
> - asking clients about their habits, values and culture, instead of making assumptions and generalisations;
> - working with the assistance of interpreters whenever necessary.

3.3 Varied Skinscapes

> The skin is both an object and means of perception. Understandings of the skin and of touch vary across cultures: the skin may be seen as social rather than individual, as porous instead of an envelope, and as knowledgeable or sentient in its own right rather than subservient to the eye or brain (i.e. cognition). These contrasting understandings have important implications for practice. (Howes, 2018, p. 225)

In the passage quoted above, pioneering sensory anthropologist David Howes reminds us that not only do touch practices vary across time and cultures, but the very understanding of the skin and its importance for knowing about the world and relating to other beings varies too. In modern Western cultures in particular, the skin is regarded as an 'envelope': something that sets one apart from others. The term 'skinship', coined by anthropologists, better illustrates the conceptions of skin found in many non-Western societies: skin is distributed and relational; it encompasses all the members of one's kin group, and sometimes non-human bodies such as animals or spirits too (Howes, 2018). For a Westerner, it is perhaps difficult to understand what 'social' or 'porous' skin (or indeed a whole porous body) means, but a simple thought experiment might run as follows: how would it affect your way of touching someone else's skin, or your experience of being touched by someone else, if you believed that doing so concerned not only the two of you but also your families, kin relations, fellow villagers, non-human beings or even the cosmos? Cynthia Sear (2020) states that we all actually were awakened to the porous nature of our bodies by the COVID-19 pandemic.

It is obvious that the elementary cultural idea of skin(ship) can sometimes be an essential factor in tactile client encounters. Since the skin or the whole body is understood in many cultures as social and relational rather than individual, the norms of interpersonal space and proper touch can extend to the client's family members or other people, most obviously in healthcare (cf. Kelly et al., 2017). In Western cultures, the individual's privacy and autonomy are highly respected values in all kinds of client work practices, including healthcare and social work, to the extent that family members may even feel excluded from information and procedures concerning the patient or client. This principle cannot be applied to all cultures. Pekka, a Finnish nurse who had worked in a Saudi Arabian hospital, described in his touch biography how the local culture differed fundamentally in this regard compared with his own background. He wrote that a family member would stay close to the patient on the ward nearly all the time, especially if the patient was the oldest male in their kinship network or was otherwise a person of very high social status. Therefore, in addition to the patient himself—Pekka was only allowed to take care of male patients—Pekka was expected to shake hands with family members as many as five times a day, and they would touch Pekka a lot in other ways too (see also Sect. 2.1.1).

The Saudi Arabian case exemplifies the concrete consequences that an understanding of skin as fundamentally relational can have for touch practices at work. Another example can be found in the case of the Filipino-Canadian patients whose interactions with nurses in Canadian hospitals were observed by Alberta Catherine Y. Pasco and her colleagues (Pasco et al., 2004). In Filipino culture, the definition of the patient extends to the family, and this shapes all communications between the patient, family members and nursing personnel. Nurses are expected to work towards the position of *hindi ibang tao* ('one of us'), which is a category of closeness in social interactions and guarantees an open and trusting relationship between professionals and patients. *Hindi ibang tao* is distinct from the more formal connectedness of *ibang tao* ('not one of us'), and it requires spending time with the patient and family, communicating care issues through family members, responding reliably and promptly to requests for nursing care and using the languages of touch, words, the gaze and food in certain ways. Filipino patients had various terms to describe different modes and qualities of touch, and they evaluated whether they were touched gently and respectfully. Touching the patient in proper ways, letting family members perform the most intimate touching tasks and communicating with the patient through family members in certain situations were all vitally important for forming an ideal care relationship.

By contrast, Cristina Douglas (2021) presents an interesting take on the constitutive power of professional touch to create new skinships that extend beyond family or kin in the conventional sense. In her study of professional touch in Scottish dementia care facilities, she describes a young nurse who said she felt close to her grandparents in Uganda when she affectionately hugged the residents. In this way, the nurse 'recreate[d] her kinship network broken by physical distance'. Douglas also reports an incident involving an older male resident called Ian. One day, on seeing Douglas holding another resident's hand, Ian asked her to hold his hand too, asking her: 'Is Mary coming today?' This led to a uniting touch between them:

From the height of his specially tailored wheelchair, he extended his hand to me – In reaching towards me, Ian not only drew me into relation, but also enabled 'the creation of worlds' […]: the creation of relations that re-invent those who get in touch. I took his hand and asked him how he was doing. I did not know how to answer that, let alone who Mary is. But, in holding hands, he initiated conversation and recreated me into the image of a familiar person. In holding hands, we had become kin. (Douglas, 2021, p. 10)

Perceptions of touch are influenced not only by conceptions of skin relations between humans but also by skin relations with other beings and the environment, which vary across cultures. According to Howes (2018), habits and meanings of touch can only be understood when considered as parts of complex *skinscapes*, that is, (dis)entanglements of human and non-human agents. Touch is often a crucial channel of contact with the natural environment and animals for people who work in primary production (horticulture, farming, herding, forestry or agriculture) or live in the countryside. However, with the constantly accelerating urbanisation and technologisation of primary production, skinscapes have changed dramatically. A typical urban skinscape, at least in rich countries, consists mainly of plain surfaces,

> **Box 3.3 Changes in European Skinscape**
>
> In her book *The deepest sense: A cultural history of touch*, Classen (2012) discusses changes in European skinscapes from the Middle Ages until today. The development of the Western 'culture of comfort' and consumption meant the 'decline of the mediaeval tactile cosmology' in which tactile contact with other humans and animals was more skin-centred than in the modern era. Industrialisation and urbanisation wrought vast changes in people's everyday lives. Modern cities gradually became crowded with immigrants with different cultural and social backgrounds and sensory practices, which caused anxiety about 'contamination' and 'contagion', especially among the middle class. This class distinguished itself from others by controlling its sensory habits and separating the home as a private sphere.
>
> New rules about cleanliness and hygiene, and other 'distancing' practices such as eating with cutlery and communicating through new media (letters, postcards and telegrams), led to a way of life where there was less and less tactile contact with the human and natural environment outside the home. Accelerated migration to cities, together with increased material standards of living and hectic rhythms of working life, have increasingly individualised our lives, and the price to be paid is often loneliness. Contamination and contagion in crowds are highly topical concerns once more, as the COVID-19 pandemic is globally changing societal structures and touch cultures in unpredictable ways.

'cold' screens and static temperatures (Howes, 2005). 'Skin knowledge' in a technologised culture focuses on haptic knowledge during the use of technological devices, while cognition is associated mainly with sight (Box 3.3).

Fundamental changes in our skinscape are moulding client work too, in a context where the term 'development' is often unquestionably equated with digitalisation. We have encountered this equation in our own work: we must provide annual reports to our university administration about how we have 'progressed in our teaching skills by adopting new digital teaching tools'—other ways of developing our teaching skills, such as through sensory skills, are not even asked about! We focus on the relation between technology and touch in client work in Chap. 4. In general, with regard to skinscapes, today's hypertechnologised way of life has caused serious trouble: we are arguably losing touch with the flesh and interacting mainly with algorithms through technological devices (Gross, 2019). For many people living in urban environments, voluntary tactile stimuli from natural elements or animals are something 'extra', even extraordinary, and need to be specially arranged. On the other hand, people increasingly keep pets in their urban homes, and activities around green plants and urban farming are becoming popular. It is also interesting to note the ever-increasing popularity of animal-assisted care, education and other forms of client work, especially in work with people with special needs. The use of animals in client work is based predominantly on the sense of touch, since touching animals provides various benefits to different client groups. Our interviews also demonstrated that professionals thought that living pets would be beneficial for residents in nursing homes, for example, as the residents would experience skin contact with them as a form of caring touch. In their touch biographies, many of our Finnish research participants considered the touch of animals to be their most stress-free, pleasant or natural form of touch. Dogs have also been introduced to mitigate healthcare professionals' stress in the workplace (Maran et al., 2022). On the other hand, the introduction of animals, especially dogs and horses, as touch therapists and communication facilitators for a growing number of clients and professionals alike is giving rise to new ethical dilemmas (see e.g. Barker & Gee, 2021).

One form of this changed skinscape can be detected in sensory medical practices, such as in the use of investigating touch. Although nurses, physiotherapists and masseurs in particular still rely on their skin knowledge when treating their clients, the medical patient's body has increasingly become an object observed from a visual distance whose internal sensory experience does not always correspond with the doctor's 'scientific' view (Box 3.4). Further, it could be claimed that professional skin knowledge and touch are racialised, ethnicised and gendered, and this is reflected in the organisation of healthcare work: the 'distant' sense of sight is associated with whiteness and maleness, while the 'near' sense of touch is associated with femaleness and ethnic 'otherness'. Thus, social distinctions and hierarchies are reproduced by the senses in working life too. An example of this is the increasing number of people of colour to be found in high-touch care and cleaning jobs (such as associate nursing and nannying) in public and domestic spheres in many Western countries. For instance, Filipino care workers are one of the biggest immigrant care worker populations in many Western countries. They are often desirable workers because of their reputation as hardworking employees who will do 'dirty' and 'demanding' work and are 'passionate' about providing care, even to older adults who are strangers to them (Lovelock & Martin, 2016).

The racialised division of labour also has long roots in the United States, where (as in Europe) 'low-touch' jobs (such as doctors' jobs) are seen as 'white' (Batnitzky & McDowell, 2011). The uneven ethnicised and racialised distribution of labour reproduces cultural discourses and meaning-makings that have a strong influence on educational practice. It has been noted in Finland, for example, that Somalian or Romany girls are much more likely to be advised to train for associate nursing than to become medical doctors. There is also a political consensus that the alarming shortage of healthcare professionals, especially in primary care, can only be resolved by an immigrant workforce from developing countries. The danger is that caring and touching abilities are expected to come from 'others' recruited abroad rather than from Western workers, which may lead to structural discrimination in education, workplace divisions and uneven pay policies.

In sum, there are remarkable individual and cultural variations in how tactile contact between humans, natural elements, animals or technological devices are

Box 3.4 Varied Sensory Orders
An interesting example of different forms of sensory knowledge about disease and healing was found by Susan J. Rasmussen (2006), who studied female healers among the semi-nomadic Tuareg people who inhabit areas of Niger and Mali. These much-respected older women diagnose diseases by palpating the patient's stomach and joints, in this way gaining knowledge about the 'imbalances' that are causing the disease, which may concern diet, marital issues or relationships with ancestors and spirits. Healing practices include the use of herbs and comforting touch in the form of skin stimulation, massage and physical support. One healer said to Rasmussen (2006, p. 61): 'Me, I [also] use barks. [But] the person who does not know touch does not know medicine'. Tuareg women emphasised that the main difference between marabouts (Muslim scholars) and themselves was that they healed by touching while the marabouts healed by writing. No doubt, Tuareg healers would consider writing and looking to be the main modes of healing in Western medicine too. A doctor looking intensely at their computer screen in the surgery seems to be detached from the embodiment of the patient, and indeed from the whole encounter.

The privileged status of sight has long historical roots in the Western sensory order, where touch has been categorised as the 'lowest' sense. Touch has been associated with animality rather than humanity and femininity rather than masculinity and has also been understood as the least 'white' sense. Plato and Hegel located touch at the lowest level in the human sensorium, on the borderline between the human and animal senses (Synnott, 1997). During the nineteenth century, the natural historian Lorenz Oken developed a racial hierarchy of the senses, in which white Europeans represented the highest category of 'eye-man', followed by the Asian 'ear-man'. Next in the hierarchy was the Native American 'nose-man', and then came the Australian 'tongue-man'. At the bottom of the scale was the African 'skin-man' (Classen, 1997).

It is worth noting that the original Aristotelian classification of five basic senses—sight, hearing, taste, smell and touch—itself varies across cultures. It makes little sense, for example, in cultures where there is a shared conception of a 'sixth' spiritual sense, or where the same nouns or verbs are used to refer to what Westerners would regard as two or more different senses. The subtlety of the verbal distinctions between sensory qualities usually reflects the intensity with which a sense is involved in everyday life (Goody, 2002; Howes, 2010). It is probable that some languages have more verbs or nouns to describe the qualities of different kinds of touch while others have far fewer. Further, we assume that the subtlety of the norms regulating touch between individuals in different social positions and with non-human beings also varies, although to our knowledge there is no cross-cultural data on this topic.

organised in people's everyday lives and work environments. The role of skin knowledge varies according to both culture and social status, including in client work. Client work is undergoing a digitalisation process whose outcomes and long-term influences are hard to predict but have already deeply remoulded work practices and body-to-body communication with clients, as we discuss in Chap. 4. From the touch point of view, client work environments can be considered to be specific skinscapes where human bodies interact not only with each other but also with different kinds of non-human bodies: computers, other technological and digital devices, manual instruments, spatial architecture, furniture etc. Although the skinscapes of client work have rapidly become technologised, we want to believe that this will not necessarily mean a lack of human touch in future client encounters. Whatever the skinscape, many work tasks cannot be performed without a human touch. The question is how that work is organised, valued and rewarded. Further, the possibility of more-than-human touch in client work also offers prospects that are worth considering from cultural and ethical viewpoints.

3.4 Gendered and Sexualised Professional Touch

Social life and sensory relations are organised through gender in many societies, including in working life. Gendered cultural norms of touch are reflected in working practices; conversely, working practices performed by gendered persons (re)produce societal structures and cultural meanings. Individuals construct their gendered professional identities in interaction with other actors in their working environments and are socialised into practices and discourses that carry gendered meanings of which the individual is not always fully aware. Socialisation into different gendered professional touching norms is one of those more or less conscious processes that still happen even in countries that officially pursue policies of gender equality in education and working life. For example, although Finland (like other Nordic countries) is celebrated as one of the world's most egalitarian countries, its labour market displays extreme gender segregation from the perspective of low-touch versus high-touch work: the care and education sectors are female, while technology is a male sector.

High-touch jobs such as nursing, childcare and preschool education are strongly gendered in other Western countries too. In northern European countries and the United States, the number of male nurses (including registered and associate nurses) varies between 5% and slightly over 10%, whereas in some southern European, Middle Eastern and African countries the percentage is very much higher. Several reasons have been offered to explain this segregation, ranging from inborn biological differences to socialisation practices and cultural stereotypes that maintain prejudices and cause entry barriers in education and the labour market. The current understanding is that although forms of production, economic structures and organisational policies have changed enormously since the early period of industrialisation, historical trends in labour segregation still persist. If we were to summarise the legacy of social expectations regarding the functional uses of touch at work, we might say that in many cultures women are socialised to form relationships and provide care through touch, while men are expected to exert control and demonstrate power and protection through touch. To some extent, this even applies to interpersonal touch in the private lives of heterosexual dyads, as indicated in some studies based on observations of behaviour in public places (see Seeman Smith et al., 2011).

In healthcare, the persistence of cultural stereotypes has been verified by several studies that consider both patients'/clients' conceptions and workers' experiences. Research has found that in Western cultures, male and female patients alike prefer the touch of female rather than male staff members. Edwards (1998) sees this preference as signifying that nurses' work is an 'extension of their role as wife and mother', which includes permission to perform intimate procedures. The traditional socialisation process through which females are taught to be nurturing and caring undoubtedly explains these attitudes. Since men are more expected to provide authority, protection or technical abilities in healthcare work—indeed, men are expected to show these abilities in working life in general—male nurses simply do not 'feel right'. This applies to Western culture, where most of the empirical studies of gender in nursing have taken place. Male nurses report that remaining for several years in an 'ordinary' nurse position arouses suspicion, especially among other males. They are expected to move rapidly up the organisation's hierarchy to management level (McDowell, 2009, pp. 175–178). Thus, working as a male nurse in your twenties is not a problem, but more than 20 years in the same job undermines a male nurse's 'true' masculinity in the eyes of other men. On the other hand, male nurses feel that their contribution to care is often devalued. Female professionals may see them as lacking competence, avoiding care tasks and creating disorder (Dahle, 2005).

Medical doctors, by contrast, are often perceived as male experts who are allowed to make diagnoses and decisions (Edwards, 1998). This gender division has historical roots. In Europe, hands-on healing methods were undertaken by women for centuries until modern medical practices became more common. While women were prohibited from attending universities, they could not acquire the new medical expertise based on visual and auditory techniques (Classen, 2012, pp. 79–80). Therefore, the profession of medicine was long reserved to males only, while women did nursing jobs. The French philosopher Bernard Andrieu and his colleagues (Andrieu et al., 2012, p. 160) state that socialisation into touch through gender is an important dimension of 'medicine as a tale of the skin'. They see touch as a 'somatechnic' for domination or accompaniment, and 'the sense of care is different if individuals have a gendered consciousness of their role and power, meaning that touching can never be a neutral experience' (Andrieu et al., 2012, p. 160).

In Chad O'Lynn and Lorretta Krautscheid's (2011) study of patients' experiences of nurses' intimate touch in the western United States, a younger male patient commented that he had found treatments performed by female nurses to be 'easy because women are like mothers and mothers do those things'. Female nurses themselves may also compare their work to their role as mothers (Routasalo & Isola, 1996). No wonder female nurses are often seen as utilising their inborn traits and competencies as caregivers—note that the term 'nursing' originates from the Latin *nutrientibus* and means suckling! Somewhat to our surprise, this gendered essentialisation of care work also emerged in our own interview with a pair of young nursing students 'Tiina' and 'Tanja', as the following extract demonstrates:

> Tiina: There are a lot more women in care work than men. I wonder how men experience the work because they probably don't have the care instinct based on evolution. I don't understand how men construct their care attitude.
> Interviewer: Nurse identity?
> Tiina: Yeah, right. Sure, men are capable of being in a relationship and expressing affection in it. But when the person changes every day and you should create a connection with them, it's a bit…
> Tanja: I agree. There are quite many male nurses, but they have their own families, they have children. Of course, not all have, and you can see the difference whether one is a father or not.
> Interviewer: Oh, you can see the difference in practical…
> Tanja: Definitely, especially in paediatric care.
> Tiina: And when it comes to student colleagues, there are more males specialising in emergency care, and they have their practical training. They are a lot more rational thinkers than 'how terrible, the patient is so in pain, what can we do?' Of course, females can also think rationally and reflect very logically about what could help and how, cause-and-effect relations, but males are somehow univocal.

These interviewees thought that having their own children helped male nurses to adopt the nurse identity as a kind of fatherly orientation to their work, although men overall tended to work more 'rationally' than their female colleagues. Male nurses' suitability for emergency or intensive care, which involve highly technological working environments, is a common belief and in line with the cultural script of masculinity. Psychiatry is still an attractive specialisation option for male nurses because of its historical nature as a form of security work with potentially aggressive patients. Although communication skills and medical treatments are much more emphasised in psychiatric nursing today than was the case a few decades ago, this work may still have associations with male guarding bodies (Dahle, 2005). Female caregivers are typically assumed to be better at providing hands-on care and dealing with the intimacy-related challenges of touching the patient naturally without the risk of sexually tinged touching.

Unlike female nurses, who are supposed to be mothering by instinct, male nurses often feel obliged to redeem their own professional credibility by carefully regulating their caring touch and exaggerating their protective or controlling touch. As a result of their analysis of numerous studies on the touch of male nurses, Martina Ann Kelly and colleagues (2017) use the metaphor of the gladiator's arena to discuss care work for male nurses. They note that both the researchers and the research participants in the studies they review often use warlike terms such as 'threatened' or 'defensive strategies' or understand their uniforms as 'armour'. Touch between a male nurse and a client appears to be emotionally charged and threatening to both parties, which they try to neutralise with various tactical manoeuvres. These include speaking disrespectfully about homosexuality and avoiding physical contact. When it comes to sexual instincts, male nurses (like male teachers, coaches, etc.) are not necessarily supposed to behave rationally at all. Male nurses tend to avoid touching female clients in particular on their own, and they are careful with their verbal expressions while touching them, whereas female professionals do not feel the same pressures (e.g. Gleeson & Higgins, 2009). In a study investigating professional touch in the UK from the nurses' point of view, one male nurse responded:

> I am just very aware of the allegations ... It's just something that I am very uncomfortable with if I would be left on my own with a female patient. (Keogh & Gleeson, 2006, p. 1173)

The ages of the professional and the client are another factor that is known to influence how cross-gender touch is experienced in nursing. When both parties are similar ages, female and male nurses and patients often feel uneasy about tactile contact with their own gender (Edwards, 1998; O'Lynn & Krautscheid, 2011). On the other hand, young female nurses may find touching elderly men to be 'risky' (see Kelly et al., 2017, p. 38). However, it should not be ignored that young male nurses may also face situations in which touching older female clients feels embarrassing. A male nurse working on a psychiatric ward for elderly patients described a strange situation:

> It was a strange feeling. Here I was, just starting my nursing career, washing this lady's private parts. She was very happy for me doing so, but I felt embarrassed, and I also realised how much power the white uniform gave you. (A Dutch nurse, quoted in Van Dongen & Riekje, 2001, p. 155)

In some cultures, cross-gender physical proximity, touch and eye contact are considered invasive rather than reassuring. In many Muslim and Hindu societies, all cross-gender touching is highly regulated, including in encounters with healthcare professionals, although practices differ. Some Muslim female patients, for example, may consider shaking hands with a male doctor to be appropriate, while others may feel that only a female-to-female handshake is acceptable. Even task-oriented touching with instruments may be experienced as sensitive, and a female patient may therefore prefer a male doctor to 'sound' the body only from the back and not from the front. On the other hand, male-to-male touch may be even more regulated than cross-gender touch in some cultures (Williams et al., 2013).

However, there are also reports that gender is a secondary issue in tactile contact for professionals and clients in different professional and cultural contexts. Patients may only be interested in whether the nurse or doctor is competent (e.g. O'Lynn & Krautscheid, 2011). Nurses may neutralise sexual connotations by explaining away the patient's behaviour through their illness or mental condition, as our own interviews indicated. In some organisations, gender may not matter much in working arrangements. Nevertheless, movements such as #metoo have had a deep impact on organisational practices. It has been acknowledged that unwanted touching is a powerful vehicle of harm, subordination and violation of people in working environments. This increased awareness of and pressure to eliminate improper behaviour, including direct harassment by touching, can be seen in the rise of equality working groups, panels and contact persons in various organisations.

The heated issue of child sexual abuse was especially foregrounded in the United States during the 1980s, when leading media outlets dubbed the problem a 'hidden epidemic'. There were estimates that hundreds of thousands of children were being abused every year, which had profound consequences for professional policies. 'By the 1990s, the role of the school as the front line of detection in the war against child abuse (in particular, child sexual abuse) had been cemented, and most new teachers are now educated about "the abused child"', as the sociologist Gordon Tait wrote in 2001. It is unclear how many children are actually abused in the school environment—some reports estimate that between fifty and seventy-five per cent of all cases are incestuous, and that ninety per cent of victims know the perpetrator. However, revelations of abuse in certain education institutions on the one hand, and an increased fear of unfounded accusations of inappropriate behaviour on the other, have led to strict no-touch policies in schools, nursery schools, day care centres, and other childcare and youth work settings. Besides the United States, decreased touching out of a fear of lawsuits has been reported in the UK, New Zealand and Scandinavia, especially in work with children (see Tainio et al., 2019; Varea et al., 2018). Indeed, many child-related settings are becoming no-touch zones because of the fear that any touch might be misunderstood or misinterpreted by a child or observing adult. Similar concerns may apply to 'infantilised' others such as students, women and old people, as Piper and Smith (2003, p. 880) state.

Alongside the overt sexualisation of touch, male teachers in general feel that they are working under constant surveillance and fear being accused of sexual harassment or abuse. This gives rise to contradictions at work, since touch is perceived as a necessary pedagogical skill for the guidance of and communication with children, who may themselves actively touch teachers and expect reciprocal touching (Tainio et al., 2019; Varea et al., 2018). Male nurses have also reported feeling anxiety in situations where female patients initiate touch (e.g. Gleeson & Higgins, 2009). In their study of touch communication between National Collegiate Athletic Association athletes and coaches in various sports, Michael J. Miller and colleagues (2007) found that male coaches expressed concern about touching female athletes. A male swimming coach commented: 'Cultural norms are almost physically stifling sometimes; there are literally a million directions you shouldn't go with touch'. Female athletes felt that in some situations, male coaches were almost *too* aware of the cultural restrictions and their caution with touch was exaggerated. As one female athlete put it:

> It's funny, I'll be trying to learn something new and it'll be obvious that he needs to touch me to show me how to do it, but I almost have to say, hey you can touch me before he'll do it. (American female athlete, quoted in Miller et al., 2007, p. 9)

Besides sports-related 'technical' touching, these researchers found that touch was an important way of enhancing mutual connection, showing appreciation and support, comforting and sharing emotions during intense events. However, male coaches, and female coaches who used male assistants, felt exposed to the public eye, which caused them some concern. As one coach said: 'I don't want people to think anything' (Miller et al., 2007, p. 10). Therefore, male coaches sometimes found especially female athletes' initiations of touch embarrassing. Conversely, a female athlete might find the touch of a male coach uncomfortable but feel pressured to endure it because it felt necessary for their mutual connection.

In our interviews with secondary school teachers, it emerged that apart from a few exceptional situations, teachers generally avoided touching their pupils under any circumstances. 'Seppo', a male teacher who we interviewed, told us that on occasions such as the delivery of school year report cards at the school's spring festival, he might ask his female students beforehand whether they wanted him to hug them when they received the cards. Interestingly, as Seppo pointed out, male pupils were not even asked the question. Perhaps male-to-male touch in this context is permeated by a 'triple stigma'—associated with the dangers of abuse, homosexuality and feminine emotionality and embodiment. Research suggests that male teachers at all education levels are more fearful than their female colleagues about touching children for any reason. This moral panic—or 'immoral panic', as Heather Piper (2014) puts it—has led some education institutions to decide not to hire male workers, and such attitudes effectively prevent men from joining the profession. It has even been speculated that teaching might become a women-only profession (Tait, 2001).

The burden of affective work under such circumstances is therefore different between male and female professionals. Male teachers, nurses and other professionals are expected to perform distancing touch and to adopt a work attitude that refrains from touching children, patients and clients. At the same time, male professionals are expected to be ready and able to use coercive or technology-mediated touch as a matter of course. Female employees, on the other hand, may be allowed more time to get used to technology-mediated touch, while also being expected to have an innate capability for nurturing touch.

Latin American, southern European and African working cultures are probably more tactile-oriented compared with 'Americanised' working cultures situated in non-contact culture areas. For example, research has indicated that Brazilian psychotherapists deem hugs and kisses to be more appropriate than do their peers in the United States (Miller et al., 2007). African patients may express the need for close tactile contact with hospital personnel (Gleeson & Higgins, 2009, p. 386). Spanish teachers touch their teenage students much more than do British teachers (Piper & Smith, 2003). In Japan, touch is seen as an essential part of some psychotherapeutic practices (Sakiyama & Koch, 2003), unlike in Western countries, where touching clients is perceived as not only risky but even shameful for psychotherapists. However, touch is becoming politicised and juridicised in contact cultures too, including in professional contexts. Valeria Varea and her colleagues (2018) studied Spanish 'pre-service' physical education teachers. They found that due to the increasing no-touch policies, touching had become a 'risky business' in schools, even in physical education, where touch had previously been regarded as normal and embedded in the profession. In Japan at the turn of the millennium, the Western 'touch panic' influenced the codification of ethical professional practices by the Japan Dance Therapy Association (Sakiyama & Koch, 2003).

Intensive regulation of the touching of children or other clients may prevent abuse or harassment. It is a fact that in the Catholic Church in particular, abuse has been a long-standing institutionalised practice and criminals have been protected. Sexual harassment is a widespread problem in numerous countries, and it concerns children as well as the adults who have been active in the #metoo movement. However, there is a growing concern that touch is being lost from all kinds of human contact, including in professional settings. In her popular science book *How to feel: The science and meaning of touch* (Subramanian, 2021, xiii), Susha Subramanian writes about the 'demonisation' of touch in American culture over the past few decades:

> Fears about lawsuits and the rise of the #metoo movement have made us avoid any interactions that might hint toward inappropriateness. Because affectionate touch tends to be reserved only for our most intimate relationships – with exceptions depending on our culture, gender, and personality – many people don't receive any. It's not yet clear whether our etiquette is protecting us or alienating us from each other.

It must also be remembered that withdrawal from touching is a strong emotional signal in many situations, not least with children and vulnerable adults. If we choose not to touch at all for fear of being misinterpreted, we are helping to deepen the epidemic of loneliness.

3.5 Complex Touch Cultures: How Do I Survive?

All individuals are born and live in a social, cultural, material and historical environment and are socialised into certain touching cultures. In the globalised world with its processes of multiculturalism, interculturalism, cross-culturalism and syncretism, touch cultures are constantly on the move: they unify and diverge in new ways. Practices and meanings of touch do vary across societies, groups and individuals, and we therefore need concepts to describe them—while nonetheless remembering that concepts such as 'Western', 'Hindu' and 'Muslim' touch cultures are abstract, generalised and artificial, and need to be constantly redefined and redivided into subcategories. In any case, most people feel they need some concepts to position their own social identities while also being encountered individually.

There are numerous necessary 'objective' touches—such as certain caring interventions, medical treatments and technical procedures—that are basically the same everywhere. Some studies also state that certain body parts, especially the hands, arms and shoulders, are universally 'neutral' body zones for touching, whereas the genital area in particular, regardless of culture, is perceived as an intimate body part where touching is allowed only for close partners or family members (e.g. Suvilehto et al., 2019). Touching 'neutral' body parts doubtless often secures the professionality of touching, but for example some nurses that we interviewed said that they also stroked their clients' cheeks, forehead or hair, or else hugged them, which many clients clearly found very pleasant. However, cultural and individual variances must be taken into account: some studies have indicated, for example, that clients may experience a professional touching their (or their child's) face, head or hair, or putting an arm around their shoulders, as too intimate (see Gleeson & Higgins, 2009; McCann & McKenna, 1993; Schneider & Patterson, 2010). Further, the technique for taking a blood sample may not vary significantly across cultures, but many of the tactile details involved in that situation can be performed in versatile ways: the professional's manner of greeting the client by touching, touching them while taking the sample, and then touching them afterwards may be different in different cultural contexts, not to mention other sensory gestures during the encounter. Therefore, the rough distinction between contact and non-contact cultures can be a useful starting point for any professional working in multicultural or cross-cultural environments.

Many of the healthcare professionals we interviewed emphasised the importance of considering 'traditional' cultural habits, especially when touching their older clients. Referring to Finnish patients, they said that maintaining an 'adequate distance' and conducting 'formal ways of greeting' were suitable behaviours. For example, it was safer to shake hands with a Finnish patient than to hug them or kiss them on the cheek, which might be interpreted as intrusive or suspicious gestures. On the other hand, all of our interviewees argued that touch should be utilised more boldly in work than is currently the case. They also wondered why touch was still so little discussed in education or the working community. They suspected that this might be explained by the 'touch-avoidant' Finnish culture, where talking about the importance of touch is interpreted as a sign of weakness and 'female nonsense'.

However, it must be remembered that touch etiquettes are nuanced, even complex, and that they depend on the respective social positions of each touching partner and the specific situation of touching. Some touch norms concern all individuals in a society, but a significant portion of those norms are gendered, at least on certain occasions and in certain places. There is notable cultural variation in expectations regarding how different genders should touch each other, especially in public spaces, and there are usually different norms concerning touch between people of the same gender and touch between different genders, as previously stated. This of course significantly impacts on how tactile encounters should take place in professional settings if we wish to be sensitive about cultural genders and sexualities. The need to arrange same-gender nurses for patients, for example, is inevitable in cultural contexts where touch across genders is highly restricted, as is the case for some Islamic and Hindu groups (see e.g. Vatandost et al., 2020; Williams et al., 2013). In the healthcare context, patients or clients in general appreciate it if they are asked whether they would prefer to be cared for by a female or male professional (O'Lynn & Krautscheid, 2011). However, gender does not necessarily matter much or at all; the professional's ethnicity or age may matter more.

On the other hand, individuals in similar social positions do not necessarily share the same touch etiquette at all—each of us has a unique family history and a subjective life history, through which we have adopted certain attachment styles and affective repertoires. Observing communications between the client and their family members and friends may also give us clues as to the kind of touch with which the client and their family members would feel comfortable, although the professional naturally plays a different role. In any case, family cultures do differ in their touch habits, which the professional can consider to the extent they feel necessary. However, sometimes the client may wish for quite a different kind of touch between themselves and the professional. They may expect the professional to keep their touch minimal, neutral or distant even if touch would be a natural channel of communication for them with their family members. Other clients may find the touch of the professional exceptionally safe—emotionally unthreatening, for example—compared with the touch of family members.

Using touch in a functionally and ethically appropriate way implies spending enough time with the client to allow the development of rapport (Dobson et al., 2002). Touch must be used cautiously, honouring the client's personal space and attuning oneself to their needs. Michael Hunter and Jim Struve (1998), who discuss the ethical use of touch in psychotherapy, suggest that this patience should especially apply to three cases: (1) when the client is not known to the nurse, (2) when the client is experiencing psychosis, and (3) when the client comes from a different cultural background. The first case is an everyday experience for numerous professionals, while the second represents a specific situation. However, besides psychotic clients, there are many other types of clients who are in extremely fragile positions, such as refugees, victims of human trafficking, and victims of violence or sexual abuse. It is self-evident that such cases pose different challenges, and the professional must find a sensitive way to encounter them by touch (or by not touching) that takes more than only cultural factors into account. As discussed in Sect. 2.6, our care worker interviewees talked about the importance of 'listening to' and 'stopping with' the client, by which they meant that they would try to perceive the unique person and their unique situation, while simultaneously being sensitive to the different social or cultural factors that might be inherent in that situation. They emphasised that listening and stopping were not only questions of time but represented a professional stance that also included being careful and sensitive with other sensory communications. All bodily gestures are equally important in professional encounters.

Professionals inevitably communicate through other multisensory gestures besides touch—and so do clients. Listening to the client means attuning oneself to these sensory languages and 'stopping' for a while to understand the client's situation and possible future. Andrieu and colleagues (2012, p. 165) talk about 'transmission of knowledge through gestures, techniques of the body and habits' in the encounter between the professional and the patient. Listening to and understanding gestures and postures that are 'expressions of the singularity of a person', kinds of 'expression of their geohistorical situation', is vitally important to the encounter, in which both bodies are moved by their mutual effects. They refer to Diane Saulnier's (1989, p. 37) study of the non-verbal behaviour of elderly patients observed by geriatric nurses:

> Movements of the head: distance, shaking, bringing together, tremor …; facial mimicry: grimace, crumpling of the face, smile, tics; movements of the eyes: seek the glance, flow of tears, closing of the eyes, fixing of an object or a person, escape of the glance, tears to the

eyes, opening of the eyelids; gestures of the hands: absence of movements, agitation of the hands, crossing of the hands, gives the hand, gripping of an object or hand, sprouting of the finger, research of the hand of looking after, withdrawal of the hand of looking after, handshake of looking after, tighten the hand, tremors, etc. (Andrieu et al., 2012, p. 165)

All these bodily messages convey valuable information about the situation of a fragile patient without using words, and valuable multisensory messages are of course not limited to those mentioned above. Non-verbal language is crucially important in all units where most of the patients are critically ill or otherwise incapable of directly expressing their needs. When one is working in strange or multicultural environments, understanding clients' tactile and multisensory behaviours requires knowledge about cultural differences too. Even in extremely sensitive situations, clients may express (or refrain from expressing) their individual needs according to cultural norms, including the 'proper' scripts for gendered behaviour. There may also be occasions where a professional should be consciously ready to act 'in spite of' evident bodily messages and sometimes also spoken words. An anxious teenager may shout and behave in an extremely dismissive way while really meaning that they are in need of a protecting touch. Further, in some situations the professional should actively look behind the evident cultural norms or stereotypes. One of us authors once attended a workshop where a nurse who worked with severely ill elderly patients told us about a moving event. She had been conducting a discussion group for patients where they had talked about their 'future hopes'—individuals in all situations orient themselves towards the future in some way. An old man had said that he wished to be hugged by someone before he died. In the workshop, we wondered whether this man would have expressed this wish at all without that specific discussion group. As a Finnish man, he might have felt too embarrassed to express his need, and his caregivers might have not expected him to have any such need.

When they are touching children, professionals in early childhood services are expected to respect the family's cultural and religious practices. If the professional considers it reasonable to deviate from those practices, permission should still be sought from the family members, and the rationale for the suggestion should be explained (Schneider & Patterson, 2010). It should also be remembered that conceptions of proper touch and interpersonal space are not limited to professional-client contacts but also extend to spaces between and among clients. Clients from different cultural backgrounds may prefer privacy arrangements in sheltered housing or hospitals for themselves or their families that feel culturally familiar to them. As illustrated in Sect. 3.3, there may be different views of natural skinscapes that appear in conceptions of individual or 'shared' bodies or skins, for example, which may influence the ways in which communications between clients and professionals succeed.

When working in a multicultural environment, one must also remember that other sensory gestures besides touch can be interpreted in very different ways compared with the professional's own cultural background. For example, in their study of non-verbal communication between health professionals and clients in the multicultural Caribbean islands, Stella Williams and colleagues (2013) found that patients from several different cultural backgrounds found direct eye contact with older male or female persons to be disrespectful. Therefore, although eye contact and handshakes are often internationally expected ways to make contact, this expectation was not a fruitful premise for professional practice in the Caribbean:

> A doctor making eye contact with an elderly patient as a symbol of respect or reassurance would be deeply misunderstood in this territory. Further, in some territories such as the Bahamas and Jamaica, students indicated that closer proximities are considered invasive rather than reassuring, and therefore care must be taken when using non-verbal skill in the doctor-patient interview. (Williams et al., 2013, p. 43)

Of course, cultural differences in sensory communication habits, including touch norms, and preferences regarding personal space may sometimes lead to extraordinary choreographies in cross-cultural communications, including in working environments. A Finnish doctor once talked at a conference about her own experience of a situation in Saudi Arabia when she reached out her hand to a male colleague. The seemingly horrified man immediately stepped two metres away to maintain the safe zone between them. A Finnish colleague of ours who used to work in a Norwegian elderly care home experienced how conceptions of personal space vary even within Scandinavia. In the Norwegian care home, it was common practice for a professional to 'sprawl' side by side with a resident in their bed if the resident felt anxious or insecure. This felt rather confusing for the Finn, because such behaviour would have been impossible in her home country. The international management psychologist Max A. Eggert (2010) describes a phenomenon called the 'cocktail dance', which can happen at diplomatic meetings with representatives from different cultures: as Asians and Arabs move forwards in body-to-body discussions, East Coast Americans and English people move backwards.

We think that professionals should not fixate on possible misunderstandings or dissonant behaviours. Although in this chapter we have stressed various cultural, social and historical factors that will inevitably shape any tactile encounter between a professional and a client, we still want to recall the universal meanings of touch. Fundamental meanings of touch extend beyond words or cultures. A gentle touch is a sign of care and affection for another human being. It concretely marks a relationship and signifies togetherness: I have noticed you and turned my body towards you. Moreover, as important as awareness of cultural and social differences may be, it must not mean a rigid adherence to stereotypes; it should simply be used as a tool for sensitivity towards different clients.

Cultural differences should never be used as an excuse for the unequal treatment of clients or the neglect of a client's obvious needs. We agree with Virve Keränen (2022), who states in the context of early childhood education that instead of asking what kind of touch is allowed and what is not, we should ask what kind of touch would convey love and respect in each situation of touching. It must also be remembered that although practices and meanings of touch are culturally regulated, every touch is a moment of *recreating* culture—an encounter to affect and be affected by. Therefore, as Keränen also reminds us, a single act of professional touch not only concerns those present in that specific touch but also makes and breaks wider networks of relations, values and attitudes in society.

3.6 Thematic Learning Tasks

3.6.1 Reflection Activities

1. Sketch your own touch biography by reflecting on the following questions:
   - What kind of touching habits did my family have? How did they seem to differ from other families or other people I met?
   - How have I touched and been touched by other people in my later life? What kind of touch is easy and pleasant for me and what difficult, unpleasant or even repulsive?
   - What kind of personal or cultural differences in touching manners have I met during the course of my life? How did they appear and feel?
2. Think about the organisation where you work now or where you worked before by considering the following questions:
   - In what kind of situations have cultural differences appeared in my daily work?
   - Did I notice gendered or sexualised meanings of touch in my work environment, and how did this affect the performance and organisation of work routines?
   - How do members of my work community respect clients' cultural differences and personal preferences in touch practices? How do we solve the problems related to differences?
   - How do we collectively discuss the challenges of different touch cultures, and what kind of mutual support we would need?
3. Put yourself in the client's shoes and assess how they may perceive your sensory communication style by thinking about the following themes:
   - What kind of touching style do I have? How does my manner probably feel to clients of different genders, ages and cultural backgrounds?
   - How do I communicate by multisensory gestures, and what kind of feedback have I received from different clients and other people?
   - What kind of culture-sensitive capabilities do I have to develop to adjust my touching style to serve the client's best interests?
4. Think about the ways you could utilise the insights introduced by this chapter by considering the following questions:
   - In what ways is my personal and cultural background likely to affect my tactile working practices?
   - How could I utilise knowledge of cultural differences better in my work?
   - What can I do with the knowledge of different attachment styles in my work?
   - What does cultural sensitivity mean in my work? How should it be taken into account in practical work and what kind of dangers might an emphasis on cultural differences pose?

3.6.2 Fieldwork

Experiences of touch in childhood are known to be tremendously important for self-image and social relations in later life. They may also notably affect professional encounters with clients, but research in this area is very limited so far. You can advance this knowledge by collecting touch biographies from your colleagues. Post a call for a collection of written or spoken touch biographies to mailing lists or social media that target your professional community. Explain in the call what you are studying, why and how, and what kind of ethical guidelines you are following. Ask the participants to choose whether they want to write their touch biographies or be interviewed on the topic by you. You can ask the participants to talk about the following themes, for example, in their biographies:

- How have I touched other people and been touched by others during my life course?
- Is it important for me to touch animals, natural objects or some materials?
- How do I feel about my lifetime experiences? What positive and negative experiences have I had?
- What kind of experiences have I had of touching clients, and how have I usually felt them?
- How would I describe the connection between my private self and my work identity in regard to my capacities and preferences of touch?

3.6.3 Case Study

Think about the following imaginary setting and figure out how to assist Adam in his project.

Adam works as a masseur and wellness instructor in his own business. He is highly regarded in his profession and well known as an expert developing touch practices on the organisational level. He has been asked to train staff at a private residential dementia care unit to educate them in using comforting touch as part of their working routines. Adam has met representatives of the company and visited the unit.

When observing the practical work, Adam notices that the unit has a formal, 'distant' and task-centred communication culture. The employees wear work uniforms and seem to use gloves in almost all the procedures which some family members of the residents have complained about. The head of the organisation explains that the residents and employees come from diverse ethnic backgrounds, and some of the reported problems may stem from this. Adam gets the impression that the chief and some employees are genuinely willing to change the prevailing communication culture, despite the evident challenges.

Your task as a client work professional and Adam's friend is to consult with Adam on how to make his collaboration project successful. What kind of advice would you give to Adam in his efforts to:

- enable the organisation to realise the strengths and weaknesses in its current communication culture and touch practices with clients?
- help the organisation develop its touch practices in a more culture-sensitive way?
- arrange workshops to help employees understand their personal relationship to touch?
- encourage the employees to find respectful and fruitful ways of using comforting touch in encounters with clients responding to touch in different ways?

References

Ahmed, S. (2004). Affective economies. *Social Text, 22*(279), 117–139.
Andersen, P. A. (2011). Tactile traditions: Cultural differences and similarities in haptic communication. In M. J. Hertenstein & S. J. Weiss (Eds.), *The handbook of touch: Neuroscience, behavioral, and health perspectives* (pp. 351–369). Springer Publishing Company.
Andrieu, B., Laloë, A.-F., & Klein, A. (2012). Touch, skin cultures and the space of medicine: The birth of biosubjective care. In M. Paterson & M. Dodge (Eds.), *Touching space, placing touch* (pp. 151–168). Routledge.
Argyle, M. (1988). *Bodily communication*. Routledge.
Barker, S. E., & Gee, N. R. (2021). Canine-assisted interventions in hospitals: Best practices for maximizing human and canine safety. *Frontiers in Veterinary Science, 8*. https://doi.org/10.3389/fvets.2021.615730
Batnitzky, A., & McDowell, L. (2011). Migration, nursing, institutional discrimination and emotional/affective labour: Ethnicity and labour stratification in the UK National Health Service. *Social & Cultural Geography, 12*(2), 181–201. https://doi.org/10.1080/14649365.2011.545142
Benedict, R. (1934). *Patterns of culture*. Mariner Books.
Bourke, J. (2009). Dismembering the male: Men's bodies, Britain and the Great War, .
Bowlby, J. (1988). *A secure base: Parent-child attachment and healthy human development*. Routledge.
Burton, J. W. (2001). *Culture and the human body*. An Anthropological Perspective.
Cherry, K. (Medically reviewed by D. Susman). (2022). *The different types of attachment styles*. Verywell mind. Retrieved 15 January 2023, from https://www.verywellmind.com/attachment-styles-2795344.
Classen, C. (1997). Foundations for an anthropology of the senses. *International Social Science Journal, 153*, 401–412.
Classen, C. (2005). Fingerprints. In C. Classen (Ed.), *The book of touch* (pp. 1–9) Berg.
Classen, C. (2012). *The deepest sense. A cultural history of touch*. University of Illinois Press.
Cranny-Francis, A. (2011). Semefulness: A social semiotics of touch. *Social Semiotics, 21*(4), 463–481.
Dahle, R. (2005). Men, bodies and nursing. In D. Morgan, B. Brandth, & E. Kvande (Eds.), *Gender, bodies and work* (pp. 127–138). Ashgate.
Davis, I., Rovers, M., & Petrella, C. (2017). Touch deprivation and counselling as healing touch. In M. Rovers, J. Malette, & M. Guirguis-Younger (Eds.), *Touch in the helping professions. Research, practice and ethics* (pp. 13–31). University of Ottawa Press.
Dibiase, R., & Gunnoe, J. (2004). Gender and culture differences in touching behavior. *The Journal of Social Psychology, 144*(1), 49–62.
Dobson, S., Upadhyaya, S., Conyers, I., & Raghavan, R. (2002). Touch in the Care of People with profound and complex needs: A review of the literature. *Journal of Intellectual Disabilities, 6*(4), 351–362.

Dolinski, D. (2010). Touch, compliance, and homophobia. *Journal of Nonverbal Behavior, 34*, 179–192.

Douglas, C. (2021). A world of touch in a no-touch pandemic. Living with Dementia in a Care Facility during COVID-19. *Anthropology in Action, 28*(1), 8–15.

Edwards, S. (1998). An anthropological interpretation of nurses' and patients' perceptions. of the use of space and touch. *Journal of Advanced Nursing, 28*(4), 809–817.

Eggert, M. A. (2010). *Brilliant body language. Impress, persuade and succeed with the power of body language*. Pearson Education.

Estabrooks, C. A., & Morse, J. M. (1992). Toward a theory of touch: The touching process as acquiring a touching style. *Journal of Advanced Nursing, 17*, 448–456.

Field, T. (2003). *Touch*. MIT Press.

Finnish Institute for Health and Welfare. (2021). *Cultural competence and cultural sensitivity*. https://thl.fi/en/web/migration-and-cultural-diversity/support-material/good-practices/cultural-competence-and-cultural-sensitivity.

Gallace, A., & Spence, C. (2010). The science of interpersonal touch: An overview. *Neuroscience and Biobehavioral Reviews, 34*(2), 246–259.

Gleeson, M., & Higgins, A. (2009). Touch in mental health nursing: An exploratory study of nurses' views and perceptions. *Journal of Psychiatric and Mental Health Nursing, 16*(4), 382–389.

Goody, J. (2002). The anthropology of senses and sensations. *La Ricerca Folklorica, 45*, 17–28.

Greenbaum, P. E., & Rosenfeld, H. W. (1980). Varieties of touching in greeting: Sequential structure and sex-related differences. *Journal of Nonverbal Behavior, 5*, 13–25.

Gross, M. (2019). Are we losing touch with our world? *Current Biology, 29*, R265–R279.

Gupta, A., & Ferguson, J. (1992). Beyond "culture": Space, identity, and the politics of difference. *Cultural Anthropology, 7*(1), 6–23.

Hall, E. T. (1963). A system for the notation of proxemic behavior. *American Anthropologist, 65*(5), 1003–1026.

Harrison, C., Jones, R. S. P., & Huws, J. C. (2012). "We're people who don't touch": Exploring clinical psychologists' perspectives on their use of touch in therapy. *Counselling Psychology Quarterly, 25*(3), 277–287.

Howes, D. (2005). Skinscapes. Embodiment, culture, and environment. In C. Classen (Ed.), *The book of touch* (pp. 27–39). Berg.

Howes, D. (2010). *Sensual relations: Engaging the senses in culture and social theory*. University of Michigan Press.

Howes, D. (2018). The skinscape: Reflections on the dermalogical turn. *Body & Society, 24*(1–2), 225–239.

Hunter, M., & Struve, J. (1998). *The ethical use of touch in psychotherapy*. Sage.

Isaksen, L. W. (2002). Toward a sociology of (gendered) disgust: Images of bodily decay and organization of care work. *Journal of Family Issues, 23*(7), 791–811.

Jakubiak, B. K., & Feeney, B. C. (2017). Affectionate touch to promote relational, psychological, and physical well-being in adulthood: A theoretical model and review of the research. *Personality and Social Psychology Review, 21*(3), 228–252.

Keller, H. (2018). Universality claim of attachment theory: Children's socioemotional development across cultures. *Proc Natl Acad Sci, 6;115(45)*, 11414–11419. https://doi.org/10.1073/pnas.1720325115. PMID: 30397121; PMCID: PMC6233114.

Kelly, M. A., Nixon, L., McClurg, C., Scherpbier, A., King, N., & Dornan, T. (2017). Experience of touch in healthcare: A meta-ethnography across the healthcare professions. *Qualitative Health Research*, 1–13. https://doi.org/10.1177/1049732317707726

Keogh, B., & Gleeson, M. (2006). Caring for female patients: The experiences of male nurses. *British Journal of Nursing, 15*(21), 1172–1175. https://doi.org/10.12968/bjon.2006.15.21.22375

Keränen, V. (2022). *Moniulotteinen kosketus päiväkodin suhteissa – kertomuksia varhaiskasvatuksen arjesta*. University of Oulu.

Kinnunen, T. (2010). 'A second youth': Pursuing happiness and respectability through cosmetic surgery in Finland. *Sociology of Health & Illness, 32*(2), 258–271.

References

Kinnunen, T. (2013). *Vahvat yksin, heikot sylityksin. Otteita suomalaisesta kosketuskulttuurista.* Kirjapaja.

Kinnunen, T., & Kolehmainen, M. (2019). Touch and affect: Analysing the archive of touch biographies. *Body & Society, 25*(1), 29–56.

Klopf, D. W., & McCroskey, J. C. (2007). Intercultural communication encounters. Pearson.

Kyrölä, K. (2014). *The weight of images. Affect, body image and fat in the media.* Routledge.

Lovelock, K., & Martin, G. (2016). Eldercare work, migrant care workers, affective care and subjective proximity. *Ethnicity & Health, 21*(4), 379–396. https://doi.org/10.1080/13557858.2015.1045407

Mandriota, M. (Medically reviewed by L. Lawrenz). (2021). *Here is how to identify your attachment style.* PsychCentral. Retrieved January 15, 2023, from https://psychcentral.com/health/4-attachment-styles-in-relationships.

Manusov, V. (2017). A cultured look at nonverbal cues. In C. Ling (Ed.), *Intercultural communication* (pp. 239–260). De Gruyter Mouton.

Maran, A. D., Capitanelli, I., Cortese, C. G., Ilesanmi, O. S., Gianino, M. M., & Chirico, F. (2022). Animal-assisted intervention and health care workers' psychological health: A systematic review of the literature. *Animals, 12*, 383. https://doi.org/10.3390/ani12030383

Mauss, M. (1936/1973). Techniques of the body. *Economy and Society, 2*(1), 70–88. https://doi.org/10.1080/03085147300000003

McCann, K., & McKenna, H. P. (1993). An examination of touch between nurses and elderly patients in a continuing care setting in Northern Ireland. *Journal of Advanced Nursing, 18*(5), 838–846.

McDowell, L. (2009). *Working bodies: Interactive service employment and workplace identities.* Wiley-Blackwell.

Mead, M. (1935). *Sex and temperament in three primitive societies.* William Morrow & Company.

Meyer, B., & Pilkonis, P. A. (2001). Attachment Style. *Psychotherapy, 38*(4), 466–472.

Miller, M. J., Franken, N., & Kiefer, K. (2007). Exploring touch communication between coaches and athletes. *Indo-Pacific Journal of Phenomenology, 7*(2), 1–13. https://doi.org/10.1080/20797222.2007.11433953

O'Lynn, C., & Krautscheid, L. (2011). 'How should I touch you?': A qualitative study of attitudes on intimate touch in nursing care. *The American Journal of Nursing, 111*(3), 24–33. https://doi.org/10.1097/10.1097/01.NAJ.0000395237.83851.79. PMID: 21346463.

Pasco, A. C. Y., Morse, J. M., & Olson, J. K. (2004). Cross-cultural relationships between nurses and Filipino Canadian patients. *Journal of Nursing Scholarship, 36*(3), 239–246.

Piper, H. (2014). Touch, fear, and child protection: Immoral panic and immoral crusade. *Power and Education, 6*(3), 229–240. https://doi.org/10.2304/power.2014.6.3.229

Piper, H., & Smith, H. (2003). 'Touch' in educational and child care settings: Dilemmas and responses. *British Educational Research Journal, 29*(6), 879–894. https://doi.org/10.1080/0141192032000137358

Rasmussen, S. J. (2006). *Those who touch. Tuareg medicine women in anthropological perspective.* Northern Illinois University Press.

Routasalo, P., & Isola, A. (1996). The right to touch and be touched. *Nursing Ethics, 3*(2), 165–176.

Sakiyama, Y., & Koch, N. (2003). Touch in dance therapy in Japan. *American Journal of Dance Therapy, 25*(2), 79–95.

Satyogi, P. (2021). Perverse economies of intimate and personal labour. *Anthropology in Action, 28*(1), 39–46. https://www.berghahnjournals.com/view/journals/aia/28/1/aia280108.xml

Saulnier, D. (1989). Les cris répétitifs. *L'infirmière Canadienne, 85*(11), 35–38.

Schneider, E. F., & Patterson, P. P. (2010). You've got that magic touch: Integrating the sense of touch into early childhood services. *Young Exceptional Children, 13*(5), 17–27. https://doi.org/10.1177/1096250610384706

Sear, C. (2020). Porous bodies. Corporeal intimacies, disgust and violence in a COVID-19 world. *Anthropology in Action, 27*(2), 73–77.

Seeman Smith, J. C., Vogel, D. L., Madon, S., & Edwards, S. R. (2011). The Counselling Psychologist, *39*(5), 764–787.

Subramanian, S. (2021). *How to feel: The science and meaning of touch.* Columbia University Press.
Suvilehto, J. T., Nummenmaa, L., Harada, T., Dunbar, R. I. M., Hari, R., Turner, R., Sadato, N., & Kitada, R. (2019). Cross-cultural similarity in relationship-specific social touching. *Proceedings of the Royal Society B, 286,* 20190467. https://doi.org/10.1098/rspb.2019.0467
Synnott, A. (1997). *The body social. Symbolism, self and society.* Routledge.
Tahhan, D. A. (2008). Depth and space in sleep: Intimacy, touch and the body in Japanese co-sleeping rituals. *Body & Society, 14*(4), 37–56.
Tainio, L., Heinonen, P., Karvonen, U., & Routarinne, S. (2019). "Siin varmaa niinku raja ylitty." Opettajien käsitykset koskettamisen normeista ja rajoista. *Sukupuolentutkimus, 32*(3), 5–23.
Tait, G. (2001). 'No Touch' policies and the Management of Risk. In A. Jones (Ed.), *Touchy subject: Teachers touching children* (pp. 39–49). University of Otago Press.
Tanner, L. (2017). *Embracing touch in dementia care: A person-Centred approach to touch and relationships.* Jessica Kingsley Publishers.
Tirkkonen, T. (2015). *Early attachment, mental well-being and development of Finnish children at preschool age. Twinship – Risk or opportunity?* University of.
Van Dongen, E., & Riekje, E. (2001). The art of touching: The culture of "body work" in nursing. *Anthropology & Medicine, 8*(2–3), 149–161.
Vatandost, S., Oshvandi, K., Ahmadi, F., & Cheraghi, F. (2020). The challenges of male nurses in the care of female patients in Iran. *International Nursing Review, 67*(2), 199–207. https://doi.org/10.1111/inr.12582. Epub 2020 Apr 20. PMID: 32314370
Wanko Keutchafo, E. L., Kerr, J., Baloyi, O. B., & Duma, S. E. (2022). Conditions influencing effective nurse nonverbal communication with hospitalized older adults in Cameroon. *Global Qualitative Nursing, 9,* 1–11.
Williams, S., Harricharan, M., & Sa, B. (2013). Nonverbal communication in a Caribbean medical school: "touch is a touchy issue". *Teaching and Learning in Medicine, 25*(1), 39–46. https://doi.org/10.1080/10401334.2012.741534. PMID: 2333089

Further Reading

Cekaite, A., & Mondada, L. (2020). *Touch in social interaction: Touch, language, and body.* Routledge.
Curtin, M. F. (2013). *Out of touch: Skin tropes and identities in Woolf, Ellison, Pynchon, and acker.* Routledge.
Harvey, E. D. (Ed.). (2003). *Sensible Flesh.* University of Pennsylvania Press.
Kearney, R. (2021). *Touch: Recovering our most vital sense.* Columbia University Press.
Paterson, M., & Dodge, M. (Eds.). (2016). *Touching space, placing touch.* Routledge.
Smith, M. M. (2007). Sensory history. Berg.

Technology-Mediated Touch

4

Abstract

This chapter introduces the main principles of technology-mediated touch in interactive client work. Mechanical tools and digital technologies both enable and hinder professionals' ability to develop physical contact with clients. Drawing on critical technology studies and the phenomenology of the body, this chapter develops a novel approach to how technology shapes tactile interactions between professionals and clients. Devices, tools and robotics expand the abilities of the working body but simultaneously shape the user's physiology, lived body and habitus. Thus, technologies are not neutral; rather, by drawing attention to themselves, they can create digital distances, even if the professional and the client are physically close to each other. We conclude the chapter with a discussion of how the COVID-19 pandemic and the digital leap that followed have revolutionised the touch cultures of various professions, generating touch deprivation issues. Due to digitalisation, touch deprivation may affect a number of groups in society.

Introduction

This chapter introduces the main principles of technology-mediated touch in interactive client work. Mechanical tools, instruments and digital technologies both enable and hinder professionals' ability to develop physical contact with clients. Drawing on critical technology studies and the phenomenology of the body, this chapter develops a novel approach to how technological tools shape tactile interactions between professionals and clients. Devices, tools and robotics expand the abilities of the working body but simultaneously shape the user's physiology, lived body and habitus. The concept of triadic touch captures the idea that technologies, tools and material objects create unpredictable affects and tensions in interactions between professionals and clients, which the professional must learn to manage. Thus, technologies are not neutral; rather, by drawing attention to themselves, they can create digital distances, even if the professional and the client are physically close to each other. However, the sensations and experiences produced by material objects are not purely negative, and the touch of material objects can be revitalising and enjoyable. We conclude the chapter with a discussion of how the COVID-19 pandemic and the digital leap that followed have revolutionised the touch cultures of various professions, generating touch deprivation issues. Due to digitalisation, touch deprivation may affect a number of groups in society.

Learning Objectives
This chapter is designed to prepare you for analysing the impacts of digitalisation and technology on touch practices at work. By reading the chapter carefully, you should be able to:

- identify the fundamental concepts and key issues of technology-mediated touch.
- explain how mechanical tools, instruments and digital technologies both enable and hinder professionals' ability to develop physical contact with clients.
- describe how technological tools shape embodiment and effect tactile interactions between a professional and a client.
- describe broad trends behind touch deprivation.

4.1 Digital Connection Is the Oxygen We Breathe

> There is almost no one with whom I regularly interact solely face to face. I spend an inordinate amount of time with digital technology. I communicate via email, use the internet in my research and teaching, use social media for teaching, read the news online and shop online. (Professor based in North America, quoted in Anderson & Ranie, 2018, p. 3)

The professor quoted above aptly describes how digital connection has become as ubiquitous in our daily lives as the oxygen we breathe. It is ever-present in all aspects of life, reshaping our social communications, including our most intimate relationships. Before the advent of the internet, personal relationships were rarely entered into without in-person interactions. By contrast, thanks to social media, many of us have friends or acquaintances with whom we are in contact almost daily online but whom we have never met in person. On the other hand, many people say that social media apps allow them to maintain daily contact with their friends and families, and that this interaction complements in-person contact rather than replacing it.

Many face-to-face services provided by professionals have been replaced by a wide variety of digital services. Because of the internet, we have access to numerous digital services via mobile apps, many of them free of charge. From our phone, with a few taps of the finger, we can order a taxi, our groceries or a takeaway—and track deliveries, receive travel updates, navigate foreign cities or get up-to-date traffic information to avoid accidents. Many people regularly use the internet to improve their well-being and education, seek entertainment, go shopping, change employment, conduct business, look for new partners or participate in civic activities. Many customer services have been digitised, especially in banking and insecure sectors. Mobile banking has transformed services to such an extent that very few people visit physical bank branches to make payment transactions. Consequently, people spend a great deal of their day online, sometimes becoming addicted to tapping and prodding their phones, seeking out those little dopamine hits by checking their tweets, posts and messages. It has become harder to take our eyes off the screen and enjoy life without our digital devices.

What does the triumph of digitalisation look like from the point of view of touch culture in working life? Will digitalisation and robotics ultimately erode professionals' ability to use touch intelligently? How can technologies be effectively advanced and utilised without compromising the importance of human touch at work?

4.2 Work Digitalisation

> I probably spend more waking hours looking at a screen than not. And this seems to be the new normal, which is a bit jarring. If you'd told me 10 years ago that this is what everyday life would be like today, I'm not sure what I'd think. (Scientist, quoted in Anderson & Ranie, 2018, p. 4)

Digital technologies and electronic information systems have become widespread in almost all sectors and workplaces, and their diffusion has had a fundamental impact on organisational structures, communications, customer interactions, business models, workflows and employment relationships. By 'work digitalisation' we mean the increasing adoption of digital technologies to revise extant organisational processes and practices from the perspective of enhanced effectiveness and efficiency (Palumbo & Cavallone, 2022). Digitalisation can take a variety of shapes, such as the increased use of personal computers and digital devices to accomplish work tasks, the robotisation and automation of organisational processes, and the adoption of wearable tools to advance professional skills and capabilities (e.g. Rajamanickam et al., 2022). Thus, almost all modern organisations rely on digitisation (the conversion of conventional work practices into digital formats) and digitalisation (the reconfiguration of organisational models and processes enabled by information and communications technologies (ICTs)), leading to increasingly complex work environments. These phenomena are related to the digital transformation of the workplace, where digital technology is utilised to reframe individual jobs and tasks, which can now also be done remotely.

The COVID-19 pandemic has accelerated companies' digital transitions across the globe. Rocco Palumbo and Mauro Cavallone (2022) state that the transformation of the work environment due to digitalisation can be conceived of as a double-edged sword. While it promotes people-centred and flexible working arrangements, it also exacerbates work-related stressors. The digital transformation of the workplace enacts an 'always-on' culture and prevents people from detaching psychologically from their work. The pervasive use of ICTs and digital tools to reconfigure individual jobs may create an extensification of work, paving the way for irregular working hours and greater time pressures. This is particularly relevant in sectors that were previously less affected by the digitalisation of organisational processes, such as education, social work and healthcare.

Digitalisation is achieving a growing relevance in healthcare, where it has been further stimulated by the barriers to access to care imposed by the COVID-19 pandemic (Kraus et al., 2021; Palumbo & Cavallone, 2022). Healthcare institutions have attempted to take advantage of digitisation to cope with the spread of the pandemic and to deliver advanced digital healthcare services, for example by implementing health consultation chatbots in their customer interfaces (Parviainen & Rantala, 2021). The goal of these healthcare chatbots is to provide patients with access to immediate medical information, recommend diagnoses at the first sign of illness and connect patients with suitable healthcare providers. Where patients used to discuss their symptoms on the phone with a nurse, now they can type a question online and get answers from a chatbot. Similarly, due to COVID-19 lockdowns, many educational institutions all over the world have started utilising digital resources to organise distance learning, although in many cases the quality of the teaching has deteriorated significantly (Barron Rodriguez et al., 2022).

The side effects of digitalisation include more routinisation of work tasks, more staring at screens and more time spent sitting still, resulting in negative feelings about the meaningfulness of work, a desensitisation of the working environment and the hindrance of social exchanges (Palumbo, 2021). Moreover, digitalisation reframes both the professional's and the client's experience, triggering a focus on technology rather than on humans and encouraging the primacy of technology over humans in the configuration of the service dynamic. From the point of view of organisations' touch cultures, another side effect is the reduction of social contact and touching in interactions between employees and customers. Overall, digitalisation recontextualises interpersonal relationships between professionals and clients, with negative impacts on mutual understanding. As Palumbo and Cavallone (2022) argue, the pervasiveness of ICTs and digital tools reduces human touching in working arrangements and makes people feel as if they are mere appendices of technologies.

Despite the fact that the use of digital tools reduces physical contact in customer interactions, physical touching between professionals and clients is unlikely to disappear completely in digital environments. Rather, technologies will shape the forms of touching. Unfortunately, there is very little empirical or theoretical research on the role of touch in digitalised and technological environments (Arcega et al., 2020; Dean et al., 2017; Parviainen et al., 2019; Pykett & Paterson, 2022). There is an almost complete absence of discussion of touch as a central part of technology-mediated interactions between professionals and clients (Parviainen & Pirhonen, 2017). A considerable amount of research has been done regarding haptics and touching in human-machine interactions (Paterson, 2007). As we mentioned in our discussion of touch research in Chap. 1, haptics and gestural research is one of the key areas of touch research. However, haptics studies is mainly concerned with the tactile perception of material objects, and it does not address touching between people where technology plays a mediating role. The reason why haptics research bypasses human-human interactions is that haptics is a branch of human-computer interaction (HCI). This multidisciplinary field of study focuses on the design of computer technology, particularly the interaction between humans (users) and computers. While initially concerned with computers, HCI has expanded to cover almost all forms of information technology design, increasingly embracing touch research as well.

The American postmodern literary critic N. Katherine Hayles has considered the empowering role of cybernetics—and thus also of HCI—in how computer science and its way of thinking about human activity, which is primarily from the perspective of information, has spread to almost all the human sciences. In her influential book *How We Became Posthuman*, Hayles (1999) critiques the way that cognition and information are given precedence over the body and materiality. In many cybernetics-influenced conceptions—notably haptics as a branch of human-machine interaction—the body is seen merely as a container for information and code. Hayles traces the social and cultural processes and practices that led to the conceptualisation of information and cognition as separate from the material that instantiates it. She argues that there is a 'cultural perception that information and materiality are conceptually distinct and that information is in some sense more essential, more important and more fundamental than materiality' (Hayles, 1999, p. 18).

Inspired by Hayles's view, we are concerned with the way in which HCI-oriented discussions address tactile feelings mainly as information related to cognition, and ignore questions about the use of power as part of technology-mediated touch, for example. In addition, HCI-oriented haptics has neglected tactile interactions between people, even though technological devices are reshaping these interactions in multiple ways. In this book, our purpose is to fill this gap by considering what forms human-machine-human interactions can take if we focus on touch sensations and feelings. Here we develop a novel approach we call 'technology-mediated touch', reworking some influential contributions concerning the senses, the body and technologies (Dreyfus, 1992; Haraway, 1985, 2003; Hayles, 1999; Ihde, 2001: Latour, 1993; Merleau-Ponty, 1989) to better articulate how digital and material technologies as well as mechanical tools and machines enable or hinder our physical touch of other beings. Taking seriously Hayles's concern that living, vulnerable bodies have been erased from contemporary cybernetics discussions, we apply phenomenological approaches to embodiment (Dreyfus, 1992; Ihde, 2001; Merleau-Ponty, 1989) alongside critical technology research (Haraway, 1985; Hayles, 1999; Latour, 1993). Phenomenological research has direct relevance to both embodiment and technology, since phenomenologists have considered how we experience our surroundings and others through artefacts, tools and technologies. Both Dreyfus (1992) and Ihde (2001) have appealed to Merleau-Ponty's work on embodiment (see Box 4.1), and their work makes special reference to technology-mediated touch, although neither of them addresses touch in the way that we approach it.

> **Box 4.1 Maurice Merleau-Ponty's Phenomenological Formulation of the Body**
> Emphasising the importance of embodiment for perception, phenomenology examines the influence of environmental factors and other people on affective and action-oriented experience (among other things). The phenomenology of the body became a rising field in the 1980s, with the French philosopher Maurice Merleau-Ponty (1908–1961) at its heart. Merleau-Ponty emphasised that the body is an incarnated consciousness that is (prereflexively) directed and open towards the world, with which the body forms an inextricable unity. Pursuing various insights offered by Edmund Husserl and Martin Heidegger, Merleau-Ponty advanced the analysis of embodied perception by combining psychology with phenomenology, laying the groundwork for modern approaches such as embodied cognition. Following Husserl's distinction between the lived body (*Leib*) and the physical body (*Körper*), the notion of the lived body captures the body from the embodied first-person perspective, whereas the physical body is an objectified, corporeal and material entity. Furthermore, following Husserl's phenomenology, Merleau-Ponty addresses the notion of motor intentionality, which concerns the lived body's intention towards objects, its directing itself towards goals and its acting in a way that enables it to make sense of a collection of disparate bodily movements, unifying them into meaningful action (Merleau-Ponty, 1989, p. 137). Thus, Merleau-Ponty treats the lived body as the perceiver, the knower and the actor. While our primary orientation to the world is an embodied relation through motor intentionality, our hand movements, gestures, touches and whole motor systems necessarily play an essential role. Our bodies are not primarily objects—either for ourselves or for others—but subjective bodies that express their feelings in their postures, movements, gestures, touches and other bodily actions. Instead of being single bodies, Merleau-Ponty emphasises, we are intercorporeally connected to others. We engage with the world mostly as embodied agents rather than as passive observers or detached minds.

4.3 Digital Proxemics: Information Technology (Dis)connecting People at Work

> The computer molds the human even as the human builds the computer. (Hayles, 1999, p. 47)

Information technology devices—especially mobile phones, laptops and tablets—are used by almost all professionals, although their use at work varies by profession and situation. The way a scientist uses a computer in their office differs from the way a nurse uses a tablet in a care home for the elderly or a surgeon uses a computer in the operating theatre. A maths teacher relies on a computer to prepare worksheets and present information to pupils in class, while a social worker checks information about the client on a tablet in a child custody situation. The increased use of computers is changing touch cultures in working life in different ways—for example, reducing the amount of touch between the professional and the client, or exposing the client to touches with objects and artefacts more often than to touches from other humans.

Researchers have identified the ongoing digitalisation as having profound effects on working conditions, such as an increase in stress ('technostress') (Bondanini et al., 2020; Dragano & Lunau, 2020) and a lack of face-to-face interaction (Bondanini et al., 2020; Brod, 1984; Palumbo & Cavallone, 2022). While the empirical evidence is inconsistent—especially in service industries such as education and healthcare—the lack of face-to-face interaction has contributed to an increase in mutual misunderstandings between professionals and clients in these sectors. Even though the digitalisation of work may lead to richer and more continuous exchanges across an organisation, bridging distance and difference, it is expected to disrupt face-to-face exchanges, including physical contact with clients, with negative implications for the quality of interpersonal relationships at work (Palumbo & Cavallone, 2022). With regard to technostress, one of the key causes of anxiety is the constant implementation of new information systems. Many professionals feel that too much time is spent processing information and data and learning new ICT skills, triggering a focus on technology rather than clients. In addition, no extra work hours are allocated for the tasks of seeking, collecting and storing information in digital systems, or for reading, interpreting and responding to emails, which all take places away from actual interactions with clients. Of course, most reforms are justified, since information systems intended for the processing of client data must meet strict requirements with regard to data security, data protection, functionality and compatibility.

Compatible systems have been used to improve the flow of information within and between units and to prevent errors and unnecessary investigations. For instance, the health and social care sectors in particular are highly dependent on electronic information systems. In hospitals, it is almost impossible to perform work without access to appointment booking systems, electronic medical records, digital image-filing and transmission systems, and the exchange of information between healthcare organisations and units. In university hospitals, simply logging into various information systems often takes up an unreasonably large part of the work shift—not to mention the amount of time spent idle due to technology and internet problems. A fault in an electronic information system can put a halt to work almost completely. Many healthcare professionals complain that not all digital technologies can be integrated into the medical system in ways that are cost-efficient, interoperable, empowering and truly usable.

Following the outbreak of the COVID-19 pandemic, the shift from physical to digital spaces was both rapid and dramatic, and this also increased technostress. Several dimensions of technostress have been identified—for example, techno-overload, techno insecurity or stress in human-machine interactions—but being isolated and working in a digital bubble can also produce anxiety. 'Digital proxemics' is an umbrella concept that covers how proximity to other people is perceived and acted upon in malleable virtual environments and digital spaces (McArthur, 2016). It is based on Edward T. Hall's (1963) notion of proxemics and its four distance zones—intimate, personal, social and public zones (see Sect. 3.2)—all of which can be included in digital proxemics. Digital proxemics investigates (among other things) how these four dimensions appear in digital communications, shaping our identities and our perceptions of others. A digital space that exemplifies all of these dimensions is the 'echo chambers' of social media. Echo chambers are social media bubbles where outsiders' voices are systematically discredited (Nguyen, 2022). Dwelling in such digital spaces for long periods, while chatting during video games and posting on social media, can twist one's opinions, alter one's perception of what others think and thus affect one's social relationships with other people.

We use the digital proxemics approach to understand tactile cultures more clearly, especially the lack of touching in digital contexts. In our approach to touch cultures, we develop two aspects of digital proxemics that are central for understanding how touch practices and physical interactions in different jobs and professions are being modified in the digital age. We call these two opposing aspects 'digital distance' and 'gathering-around' technologies. By digital distance, we mean the zone between people who are physically present but not communicating with each other because they are on the internet, chatting on the phone, or using other technologies or apps. A digital distance zone is maintained between people when they are communicating with something or someone through the internet, a phone etc. while remaining in physical proximity with the people around them. Gathering-around technologies (e.g. mobile phones) can produce social, personal or intimate zones between people so that the use of devices connects and activates working or playing together. In what follows, we take a closer look at how digital distance and gathering-around technologies manifest themselves between the professional and the client.

According to our interview findings, many professionals feel they have less and less time to encounter their clients face to face. Often, digital devices need to be used in the presence of customers, patients and students, forcing professionals into the digital distance zone and making them ignore their clients unintentionally. The client perceives the use of the equipment as overriding their own needs and as rude behaviour, even though the use of the equipment is a necessary part of the expert's work. When we interviewed nurses about their opinions regarding the impact of digital technology on their work, many of them said it had a negative influence on their interactions with clients. The use of technologies had sometimes even prevented the establishment of tactile contact with the client because the professional had to focus on adjusting the devices. While the nurse would sit next to the client during a home visit, part of their work time would be spent typing up client information. While writing on a tablet, the nurses felt that they were not fully present to the client which they saw as morally problematic—the client anyway pays for all the visiting time. We suggest that this type of interaction with clients concretises the idea of digital distance. The nurse and the client are physically present, but the use of digital devices builds up the digital distance zone: they cannot communicate with each other because the nurse is on the internet.

The increased digital distance between professional and client can also cause unexpected conflicts in the interaction (see Haddad et al., 2019). For instance, schools have moved from face-to-face interaction to electronic systems, through which parents are informed about issues related to the child's school day and schedule, and about school activities more generally. Teachers and parents communicate with each other in words and by writing online. The most widely used teaching and learning platform in Finland is Wilma, which parents and teachers use for mutual e-communication. Many teachers feel that parents' email messages have become harsher and more demanding than was previously the case. In an interview with the newspaper *Helsingin Sanomat*, one primary schoolteacher said:

> They [parents] interfere with everything we do, question it and demand justifications. For example, when trips are being taken, which always makes the teacher busier than normal, they slow things down by asking for explanations while spoiling the teacher's enthusiasm about going on the trip. As a result, there are no excursions at all, because the teacher can't handle the flood of questions. Easier to stay in school and not do any extras. (Finnish schoolteacher, quoted in Kurki, 2022)

As the threatening tone of these parents' messages suggests, it is easier to make threats and demands in writing online than it would be in a face-to-face conversation. Sometimes a simple poor choice of words can lead to misinterpretations and spark unnecessary conflicts between teachers and parents. A written message often requires softer and more polite wording than would a face-to-face interaction to ensure that the recipient does not interpret the text as an insult or attack. Attention has long been paid to the polite wording of emails in working life, but it is easy to forget its importance if one is writing in a hurry or at midnight. Sometimes carelessly written electronic messages can escalate into larger conflicts if the rage and injury that has arisen within one's digital bubble cannot be dealt with.

However, it would be dubious to argue that the use of information technology merely reduces face-to-face encounters or increases tensions and misunderstandings between people at work. The use of mobile devices can also promote and intensify interactions in face-to-face encounters with clients, patients or students. Mobile phones and other mobile devices are used in daily practice, sometimes quite creatively. 'Eero', a home care nurse, told us how he had solved a communication problem with an elderly client who spoke only Russian. The client did not understand the home care nurse's questions in Finnish. So Eero picked up his mobile phone, typed his Finnish question into Google Translate and showed the client the Russian translation. The client finally understood what the Finnish-speaking nurse meant. Eero also said he had used Finnish YouTube music videos with an elderly patient who enjoyed singing hymns with others. While caring for the client during his home visits, Eero would play hymns on YouTube with which the client would sing along. According to Eero, the client obviously enjoyed the situation, which also created a pleasant atmosphere for the treatment.

Professor Camille Baker (2019), who specialises in interactive and immersive arts technologies, explores new forms of artistic expression that have emerged since the onset of the smartphone. She suggests that smartphones can strengthen some connections thanks to their potential to intensify embodied presence, liveness and affects between people. Baker demonstrates how people have repurposed the smartphone, transforming it from a mere voice-and-text communication device and turning it into a new collaborative medium—a fully visual, synesthetic, interactive and performative tool for deeper expression and social change.

Inspired by Baker's research, we suggest that mobiles and tablets can be used as gathering-around technologies, by which we refer to the ways in which some professionals use mobiles and tablets to develop new connections with clients and patients. In a way, mobiles and tablets can be seen as replacing the campfires around which people have gathered for millennia to tell stories and be together. At their best, gathering-around technologies bring people together, create new connections between them and provide new contexts for touching, chatting and being present with others. For example, reading and looking at pictures on a tablet can provide a moment for a nursery schoolchild to sit on a caregiver's lap. Similarly, the use of technical devices in the classroom can bring students and schoolteachers closer together by generating new kinds of interaction. A tablet shared between students can also promote supportive and creative interactions and the joint acquisition of information to solve lesson tasks.

But while gathering-around technologies can offer new forms of interaction between professionals and clients, they do not replace work tasks that require the professional's physical interaction, presence and human touch. Mobile phones and tablets are of no use to a nurse who needs to walk a client to the bathroom or assist them with toileting. Nor can information technology help a nurse to change a dressing, or to pick out an item of clothing from the patient's wardrobe and help them put it on. With the help of gathering-around technology alone, it is also difficult to replace the interaction between teachers and students in school. The teacher is not just an expert in teaching, but a source of mental and affective refuge who can comfort a crying student or resolve disputes between students. To ensure a safe environment, the teacher's physical presence in the school cannot be outsourced to technology.

4.4 Touching with and Through Technological Tools

> Once the stick has become a familiar instrument, the world of feelable things recedes and now begins, not at the outer skin of the hand, but at the end of the stick […]. The pressure on the hand and the stick are no longer given; the stick is no longer an object perceived by the blind man, but an instrument *with* which he perceives. (Merleau-Ponty, 1989, p. 152)

As we mentioned in Sect. 4.1, there is little research on how professionals touch their clients when material objects, tools and devices are involved in the tactile event. Although this seems to be a crucial issue for professional ethics too, there is scant literature on the topic (see Stokes & Palmer, 2020). We have called this missing research topic 'technology-mediated touch': it concerns how technology modifies and shapes the touch experience between the professional and the client. Technology-mediated touch can be considered a key dimension of contemporary interactive client work in many branches of the service economy, including education, security, healthcare and social work. For instance, in the healthcare sector, various technological tools and instruments are part of interactive client work, including material tools (e.g. wipes, hypodermic needles), analogic machines (e.g. massage tables, hospital beds), digital devices (e.g. dialysis machines, ventilators) and more recently artificial intelligence (AI)-operated devices (e.g. robotic assistants). Indeed, it is almost impossible to examine touch in the work of health professionals without considering how the professional touches the patient in and through technological tools.

Phenomenology is a particularly useful approach to detect the often-invisible embodied codes of touching practices with technological tools. Merleau-Ponty spoke not about technological devices, but about mechanical tools as extensions of the body. In the extract quoted above, he describes how a blind man uses a cane as if it were an extension of his body and senses. The blind man's sense of touch in a way continues into the instrument, up to the end of the instrument. For blind and visually impaired people, a cane may be a vital, constantly used aid that allows them to move around on a daily basis. In a way, the blind person palpates the environment with the cane, even though the cane itself has no feeling and does not come to life. Similarly, the instruments used in the work of many professionals often turn into organic extensions of the professional's body. For example, a skilled barber uses scissors and a comb simultaneously as an extension of their hands while cutting their client's hair.

Deborah Lupton (2013, p. 400) argues, however, that bodies do not always intermesh smoothly or seamlessly with technology. There are sometimes disjunctions between bodies and objects, especially with tools and technologies that require the use of physical force (such as rickshaws) or are poorly ergonomically designed. But regardless of whether the object merges seamlessly with the body or instead forces the body to struggle to coordinate its use, work with technologies always shapes the user's body, and at worst can permanently damage the joints and bones. Office workers who sit staring at computer screens for long periods may suffer from chronic back and neck pain as well as tendonitis. The coordination of the body gradually adapts to the device or instrument as the body becomes accustomed to the actions involved in the device's use (Crossley, 2007). Using an instrument not only modifies one's physical movements and cognition but also generates a special kind of habitus that is closely related to one's professional identity and work culture. When an office worker sits and stares at a computer screen, they do it in their own characteristic style. When a beautician plucks a client's eyebrows, they do so in the way they have been trained, but at the same time they bring their own style and habitus to their gestures. Ways of using simple instruments such as tweezers or scissors can be very diverse, and so the touch conveyed to the client by these embodied practices also varies.

Habitus refers to a relatively enduring set of dispositions that emerges based on an individual's activity in certain environments. It is a comprehensive set of internalised tendencies—not just techniques of the lived body, but also taken-for-granted worldviews and problem-solving strategies. As habitus is constituted by various physical and mental conditions, including socio-economic conditions, it is a mechanism that connects individual practices with technological conditions (Bourdieu, 1990; Bourdieu & Wacquant, 1992). Thus, lived bodies develop their own routines and practices, based on their own educational backgrounds and life histories, in order to merge with the functions of technology. For example, although basic nurses are trained in similar methods for lifting patients, they will each develop their own habitus due to their many mental and physical differences.

The work of practical nurses is considered to be especially physically hard, despite the aids available to assist them. Many nurses think that the new care robots may make it easier to lift and turn patients. At the same time, however, they consider that transferring a patient by robot is not the same as lifting them with the support of mechanical aids. Hanna, a nurse in geriatric ward, described the transfer of patients from bed to wheelchair. During such transfers, the patient is held securely, supported and touched in ways that would not be possible if the transfer were a purely mechanical operation. Lifting involves intimacy and caring contact, which a machine cannot provide. Hanna wondered if such a patient would be 'touched at the same time' and be 'in contact with someone' even for a short time. She thought that a 'cold' machine could not convey the same supportive feeling as a human could:

> Contact through touch between people cannot be replaced. Therefore, the robot reminds me of cold machinery because of the material it is made of. I wonder if it has some padding and warm surfaces, I do not know. (Hanna, Finnish nurse)

Instead of physical strength, many nurses use their own body weight to support patients during transfers by utilising the technique of kinesthetics (Box 2.3). Although it is based on coordinating the movements of nurse and patient, a similar relationship can be developed for the handling of instruments and tools: the instruments can feel as if they are 'sitting' in one's hands. Ergonomically well-designed devices and aids promote work practices in which professionals experience these devices as comfortable and safe, without causing excessive physical strain on the body. However, there are large individual variations, so good design alone is not the only solution to develop suitable work practices. The introduction of new technical equipment always requires experimentation to find proper ways of working. Getting used to working with new equipment always takes time. The more familiar the practices become to the professionals, the less they need to focus on the tools or work tasks themselves. This has been described as tacit or embodied knowledge generated through practices using tools and mechanical instruments.

The capacity to handle objects skilfully is frequently deemed a 'lower' cortical function than mental activities such as linguistic or mathematical reasoning (Piaget, 1970). In phenomenology, by contrast, the body's movement and kinaesthesia are seen as much more essential to human intelligence, and as requiring a special attention to embodied activity (Sheets-Johnstone, 1999; see Box 4.1). In phenomenological approaches, the body's motility is seen as a source of intelligence—consider, for example, the manner in which the body explores its world, creates new artefacts, and inherently makes sense of the world by solving problems and modifying materials. Merleau-Ponty (1989) states that the human body's orientation in the world does not require representations of the situation created by the mind; rather, we are able to solve many practical problems in everyday life by using our kinaesthetic intelligence

> **Box 4.2 Don Ihde's Four Basic Forms of Technological Mediation**
> Don Ihde (born 1934) is an American philosopher of science and technology. Ihde (1979, 2001) has applied the theoretical concepts of phenomenology to analyse technology, and specifically the relations between humans and technological artefacts. Ihde (1990) argues that embodiment can never be separated from technology. According to him, nearly all human perceptions and actions are mediated by technological devices, and he advances the notion of human-technological associations. The backbone of Ihde's (1990) phenomenology consists of four basic forms of technological mediation: embodiment relations, hermeneutic relations, alterity relations and background relations. Embodiment relations are those where our perception is reshaped through a device. Glasses, for example, become a part of our perceptual experience, being transparent in use. Similarly, many of the devices that professionals use, such as the headphones worn by boom operators during film-making, easily become part of their bodies. Hermeneutic relations are those where we evaluate something by using technology. For instance, by looking at the weather app on a mobile phone, we can evaluate what to wear when we go out. Alterity relations refer to situations where we relate to technical devices in ways that are similar to the ways in which we relate to other humans. For example, some users tend to relate to Siri as if it were a person. Lastly, background relations refer to technologies that make up our environmental context, such as refrigerators and air conditioners.

'on the move'. Likewise, technology-mediated touch at work cannot be cultivated unless professionals have the space to experiment and practise different ways of touching.

Following in the footsteps of Merleau-Ponty, we can conclude that many of the technologies we use on a daily basis fundamentally reshape our bodies and perceptions, forming intelligent extensions of our bodies. Consequently, the tools and instruments used by professionals in client work require not just sophisticated movement but also constant observation and monitoring of both the client's feelings and the devices themselves. In a hospital, digital devices such as dialysis machines and ventilators need a highly trained nurse to monitor their operation and respond to their alarms while also taking care of patients' well-being. To invoke Ihde's (1990) conceptualisation, this is a hermeneutic relation (see Box 4.2). Although digital devices have automated some of the work of healthcare professionals, their use requires professionals to be able to interpret feedback from gauges and sensors, and to combine motor and multimodal sensory activity with cognitive reasoning. When accurate cognitive reasoning with different metrics must be simultaneously combined with embodied and interactive work with patients, this places many further burdens on professionals compared with physical labour or cognitive work alone.

So far, we have highlighted that professionals should recognise how they are touching the client with and through technical tools. However, it is worth remembering that all kinds of physical device can erect visible or invisible barriers to the creation of a relationship between the professional and the client. In nursing, for instance, large hospital trolleys, or devices placed on beds or desktops, can become physical barriers during the provision of care or consultations to patients. When nurses are working in front of monitors or on mobile computers, these physical barriers can impact on the quality of interpersonal relationships. They can constitute distractions to the nurse even before the nurse has developed a therapeutic relationship with the patient. To gain a deeper understanding of technology-mediated touch, it is important to take a closer look at the active role played by material objects in the mediation of touch between professionals and clients.

4.5 Triadic Touch: Technologies as Actors in Client Interactions

Many of the technical procedures conducted in hospitals, health clinics and doctor's surgeries are frightening to patients. Hard, sharp, pointed tools and equipment sometimes produce physical pain. The visual appearance of a cold, technical contraption or a complicated-looking device can be appalling in and of itself, and uncertainty about its use or function can easily give rise to fear. Technological devices and instruments are also associated with the idea of restricted movement. The prospect of some scans and procedures can be so distressing that the mere sight of a probe or a dentist's chair produces a twinge of pain. Even making a dental appointment or thinking about a blood test can be stressful. The nurses we interviewed highlighted a problem related to staff shortages in this context. Sometimes a client would have to be held down while the nurse takes a blood sample, and in some cases it would take three nurses to complete the task. Healthcare professionals often do not know enough about their patients' backgrounds to understand why some of them found certain situations so distressing. In extreme situations it might even be necessary to consider abandoning the procedure altogether and do 'just the minimum', as one interviewee put it.

In most cases, healthcare professionals rely on client data retrieved from information systems, and technical equipment is essential in the healthcare sector in general. Without such systems and equipment, professionals cannot do their jobs and help their clients. Indeed, it would be misleading to focus only on how the professional touches the client with physical instruments, because devices and information technologies constitute a complex data network. When a cannula or catheter is inserted into the patient's body, both nurse and patient are connected to an extensive network of instruments and devices (see Box 4.3) that are involved in the procedure. Technologies have their own kinds of touch and impact on human beings; they too are agents or actors. To understand technologies as actors, we can investigate the triadic relationship between clients, professionals and technology.

Much has been said by previous researchers regarding the dyadic relationship between the professional and the client, but technology has wrought major changes in

> **Box 4.3 Cannulisation as an Example of a Triadic Relationship**
> For hospital patients, the insertion of a drug cannula is an everyday care procedure for which nurses are responsible. The cannula forms a complex technological network where technology-mediated touch and the triadic relationship between the material technology, the patient and the professional are central. A complete set of technological aids is involved in the connection of the cannula: hand sanitiser, protective gloves, cleaning cloth, 70% alcohol for skin-cleansing, injection needle, dressing and tape, cannula-connected tubing and taps, drip bag and drip stand for the drugs, and containers for the waste. All of the material equipment and its hygienic maintenance and handling require support staff and effective hospital logistics and infrastructure, including electricity and water supply. As a result, the patient is touched not only by the nurse but by a number of different material actors. In addition to material and technical aids, information technology and software are an integral part of the treatment process, as the patient's electronic treatment report records observations of the cannula and changes to the injection site. From the nurse's point of view, the nature of the treatment is guided by strict hygiene regulations and patient safety, but physical touch plays an important role in the procedure's success. Prior to the procedure, the nurse must be able to reassure the patient through touch and conversation so that an atmosphere of trust and security is created. The nurse monitors and anticipates the client's mood, reassuring the patient—for example, lightly touching their arm or shoulder and assuring them that the nurse will do their best to minimise any pain. In their work, nurses gradually learn to recognise how different patients manifest tension and fear in treatment situations. They learn to find appropriate ways to calm patients. The insertion of the cannula itself can be considered a task-focused touch, but both communicative contact and caring touch with the patient are required before the cannula is inserted.

this relationship (see Scott & Purves, 1996). The triadic framework suggests that the third party in such relationships—that is, technologies, tools, material artefacts and information—is no less a part of the interaction dynamic than the humans involved. As the use of technologies has increased, it is important to consider all three interacting agents when we are investigating professional-client relationships. Instead of a single technology or device, we are surrounded and connected by a multitude of devices, simply because most digital devices need the internet to function. In many work environments, digital devices and instruments are optimally arranged to enable the employee to reach the device and connect it to other equipment if necessary. For instance, for a surgeon in an operating theatre, instruments, equipment and specialist colleagues are not a set of externally related objects, but a meaningful, cohesive entity whose joint efforts can lead to a successful operation.

Jaana Parviainen and Jari Pirhonen's (2017) formulation of the triadic relationship stems from the actor-network theory (ANT) developed by the French philosopher and sociologist Bruno Latour (1993) together with his colleagues John Law and Michel Callon. According to ANT, human and non-human actors form functional entities whereby, for example, technological devices and other material objects play an active role in interactions. Of course, devices and objects lack intentionality and autonomy, but material objects often have their own character, and this makes them beings that affect the situation. Consider the example of school and how a teacher uses material objects to concretise what is being taught. In science teaching, students are often allowed to touch material samples related to the identification of rock types or plant species because images alone are not enough to fully convey their nature. Students need to explore these samples with their hands, to touch their texture, surface, weight and density, in order to understand them as part of nature and the ecosystem. The students learn by palpation, even though school curriculums emphasise the importance of audio-visual and reading comprehension above all for learning. There are also many unintentional material features associated with teaching and learning in schools that are remembered as part of one's education. The squeak of chalk on a blackboard evokes unpleasant physical sensations. A chalk stick cannot function autonomously, yet the mere memory of its squeak has the power to produce goose bumps. John Law and Vicky Singleton (2013) sum up ANT as follows:

Perhaps, then, ANT isn't a theory. Perhaps it is better thought of: as a sensibility to the materiality, relationality and uncertainty of practices; as a way of asking how it is that people and animals and objects get assembled in those practices; and as a way of mapping the relations of practice. This is how it works in the world.

The core of ANT is the principle of radical symmetry between human and non-human actors, which dissolves the modernist demarcation between living, consciously acting subjects on one hand and merely instrumental, insentient objects on the other. However, ANT has been criticised for failing to accommodate the corporeal capacities of humans, neglecting the affective capabilities of non-human actors and ignoring the role of unexpected events in networks (Müller & Schur, 2016; Thrift, 2000). In addition, ANT does not presume any power relations between actors with regard to gender or other social hierarchies, as many feminist scholars have argued (Haraway, 1997, p. 58; Wajcman, 2004, p. 39). When the question 'who touches?' is thus expanded into the question 'what touches?', it is relevant to ask: can non-living objects touch at all (Harbers, 2005, p. 15)? More importantly, can they be held accountable for their actions? Although there has recently been intense debate about the autonomy and responsibility of robots, the basic premise of professional ethics remains that the proper use of equipment and material objects is the responsibility of the professional.

Further, from the perspective of professional ethics, it is important to consider how professionals learn to handle triadic relationships in their interactions with clients. We assume that a triadic relationship requires the professional to 'stretch' and extend their own human contact and presence 'beyond' the equipment and devices. Unfortunately, the more technologised work environments become, the more professionals need to be able to take action that will soften the clients' alienated experiences of technology. Employees must act as buffers between technological equipment and clients. Since the professional is ultimately responsible for the interaction in the triadic relationship, they usually turn to spoken language to warn the client about the pain an instrument will cause—for example, during a needle injection.

Following Ihde's (1990) notion of hermeneutic relations (Box 4.2), it is important for professionals to seek to evaluate clients' experiences of the touch of material objects and instruments, and to strive to produce as pleasant feelings as possible. Professionals should anticipate various measures by describing in advance the tactile sensations the materials will cause, such as when a beautician announces that a damp cloth may feel cool before they wipe the client's face. In many situations, this verbal softening of technology-mediated touch can also be combined with a soothing and comforting touch. The professional can ease the client's tactile experience of instruments and materials that might be intimidating or surprising, and they can show the client that they recognise them as a knowledgeable fellow human and not as an object of the action. A friendly word, a warm tone, calm movements, a smile and a pat on the shoulder express empathy for the client and establish that the professional is not causing unpleasant feelings for the customer intentionally.

Sometimes, professionals use talk to try to get the client to think about something other than the situation at hand. For instance, nurses may divert the patient's attention from the site of pain by talking about the weather or some other everyday thing, to reduce the unpleasant feeling. For healthcare professionals, safety-related factors are important during the performance of treatment procedures. The aim is to use the equipment and aids in such a way that they injure neither the client nor the professional. For some patients, the fear of pain may be greater than the pain itself, as our interviewees told us. They thought that in those cases, the client would appreciate a 'reasonable' professional approach to the situation which may mean concentrating on explaining technical facts of the treatment.

Discussing touch merely in the context of a dyadic relationship between the professional and the client ignores how material objects and technologies work not only on the individual (micro) level but also on the organisational (meso) level. On the organisational level, for example, a cannula forms a complex technological network that requires access to a patient information system alongside many other direct and indirect technologies, including electricity generated by the power grid and the sorting and transporting of hospital waste. Essentially, the main point of addressing triadic touch is to identify non-human agents and their agency within organisational structures of work. While non-living material objects such as injection needles, chalk sticks or wet wipes—or humanoid robots—are not accountable for their actions, their actions are nonetheless influential and provide a network of causes and consequences.

We emphasise that material objects are never neutral; rather, many affective properties are associated with them—for example, fear is associated with the equipment used by dentists, whereas pleasure may be associated with lying down on a masseur's table. In triadic relationships, objects have the power to influence the relationship between the professional and the client. Instead of emphasising only the social connection between professional and client, it is also important to recognise the affects that material objects produce in client work.

4.6   Work Automation, Cyborgs and Robotic Touch

> Through the robot monitor, the entire 3D world opens up to the surgeon. The operation is performed with very thin instruments. The view is extremely accurate in its impression of depth, as if it were from the cockpit of an aircraft. (Antti, Finnish surgeon, quoted in HUS, 2021)

There has been much discussion recently about how the proliferation of AI and robotics is affecting work and changing its content in various professions (Frey & Osborne, 2017). By AI we mean the use of mathematical algorithms to carry out tasks that would otherwise require human effort and intelligence (De Saint Laurent, 2018). Devices that are used for reasoning, problem-solving, making judgements and plans, communicating natural languages and devising travel routes, as well as simulations, voice recognition and strategic web-based interactive games, are all examples of the use of AI and big data (Bali et al., 2019).

The surgical platform described by the surgeon we quote above is a typical device that utilises AI and robotics. The new generation of four-handed surgical robots can be used to operate on patients for whom large-scale open surgery is out of the question. Robot-assisted surgery does not require long incisions, making recovery times faster. The camera technology used by the robot provides visibility in places that are difficult to see with standard technology. A new kind of robotic medicine also makes it possible to perform remote surgery if necessary, and the patient can even be on the other side of the world from the surgeon. Some hospitals that use surgical robots collaborate with hospitals in other countries to plan joint surgical operations at a distance.

The surgical robot is related to the surgeon's motor and sensorimotor activity, so it can be considered a bodily extension. When a bodily extension becomes so necessary that the body's functionality would be decisively changed or reduced without it, it is usually referred to as an organic or inorganic prosthesis or implant. Inorganic prostheses may be removable, portable or wearable digital or material objects. According to Donna Haraway (1985), humans' physical attachments to even the most basic technologies have already made us cyborgs. A human with an artificial cardiac pacemaker or cochlear implants can be considered a cyborg, since these devices are combined with the body's own biological feedback. Modifications such as contact lenses, hearing aids, smartphones or intraocular lenses are also examples where humans are fitted with technology to enhance their biological capabilities. Moreover, exoskeletons are essentially wearable cyborgs. They were developed to allow people with spinal cord injuries and muscular dystrophy to regain their movement and strengthen their nerves and muscles. Nowadays, lighter exoskeletons for the upper or lower body can be used to support physical work with the joints, powered by small electric motors that serve as mechanical muscles.

4.6 Work Automation, Cyborgs and Robotic Touch

A cyborg can be understood as a combination of the cybernetic and the organic, with both organic and biomechatronic body parts. This concept, which for the most part had previously been used in science fiction, gained scholarly traction thanks to Haraway's celebrated work. During the 1980s, Haraway used the figure of the cyborg to urge feminists to move beyond dichotomies between human and machine, nature and culture, and physical and non-physical. Throughout her work, Haraway highlights how non-human living beings and non-living entities (e.g. technologies) shape humans and in particular reshape our notions of subjectivity, identity and gender. Broadening her focus from cyborgs to 'companion species' in *The Companion Species Manifesto* (2003), she argues that companion species can encompass not only living beings (e.g. dogs or bacteria) but also inanimate beings (e.g. mobile phones or prostheses). She uses her father's wheelchair as an example of an inanimate companion species (Haraway, 2003, p. 167): her father would quite literally not have been the man he was without his physical aid. Through this example, Haraway shows that instruments are active agents whose role in everyday life is considerable. But although technologies and aids can activate us, they also tend to routinise and automate bodily activities. In some cases, automation makes previous human functions unnecessary, leaving people to simply monitor their delivery.

Automation in the work context describes a wide range of technologies that reduce human cognitive and physical interventions in work processes. With industrial robots, the employee's work task is mainly to monitor the operation of the machine, maintain it as necessary and update its software. While industrial and logistical robots have automated some tasks that require physical work, surgical robots have made work that requires manual precision easier for surgeons. For instance, a four-handed surgical robot can perform demanding lung, thymus and oesophageal surgery. Although the surgeon must undergo lengthy training to learn how to use the robot, after a few months their body and way of working become part of the robot's functionality. From the point of view of touch, the use of such new technologies does not only change working practices. Another possible consequence is that the touch might become completely transparent to the surgeon, who may 'forget' that they are 'touching' a patient and instead orient themselves to the surgical operation primarily as a technical problem-solving task. If the surgeon gets used to the robot, they may begin to feel that operations without surgical robots are awkward or weird, because the surgeon's entire sensorimotor system will have become used to this technology. According to Ihde's (1990) formulation of embodiment relations, technological functions can become transparent to us in such a way that we understand their impact on the end result only when they are absent (Box 4.2).

When conducting surgical operations across large distances, doctors are able to touch the patient at a distance through visual-haptic technology. During an operation, only the doctor has haptic sensation, since the patient is anaesthetised; thus, the patient does not feel the technologically mediated touch until afterwards, when they many experience it as pain or relief. Surgical teleoperations entail the ability to conduct procedures with objects through digital devices over large distances, but surgeons still need to have something close at hand. The production of these tangible presences through artificial means collapses distance and makes an extremely distant patient immediately present, actually manipulable or graspable (Paterson, 2007). For the most part, haptic models of virtual objects accompany visual representations on a screen so that the surgeon can both see and feel the object simultaneously, the haptic sensation confirming the visual impression or vice versa.

Surgical robotics is an example of automation that requires a high level of expertise from a professional. However, in many industrial and service sectors, some work tasks previously regarded as routine and as demanding low-skill competence have been automated with new types of machines and robots. The development of automation in healthcare, for example, includes patient enrolment machines in large treatment units, robotic drug delivery in home care and the introduction of transport robots in hospitals. When a client logs into a self-service machine at a health centre or hospital, the information about the login is automatically transferred to the patient information system. Doctors and nurses are informed that the patient is waiting to be admitted to the clinic. Some hospitals have introduced transport robots that move hospital supplies, patient clothing and bedding from one location to another. This recalls Ihde's (1990) notion of alterity relations whereby devices can become 'co-workers' or 'assistants' without which it would be difficult to cope with certain tasks (see Box 4.2). Relating to a technical device as a co-worker requires the device to evoke the sense of a living being. Even if the device is not emotionally close, it is perceived as essential to the work. This means that professionals organise their own work tasks in the expectation that the machine will work smoothly 24/7. Robotics can reduce the workload of manual labour, but at the same time the use of robots leads to staff reductions, with robots rather than people moving along the hospital corridors. This brand new environment is not simply a by-product of technological development but the result of a political and ethical policy with far-reaching consequences, including for the kinds of interaction that professionals can create with their clients.

Robotics is also coming to home care, as exemplified by the drug delivery robots. The nurse collects the medicine bag from the pharmacy and refills the delivery robot as necessary. When its supplies are running low, the robot sends the nurse a refill reminder. The nurse does not have to visit the client physically on a daily or even weekly basis, but can keep in touch with the client via video calls, for example. It is believed that robotics can save on home care costs as it reduces nurses' travel time to clients. However, the reduction in home visits runs the risk that elderly clients may be left for days with no human contact. This in turn means fewer and fewer opportunities for human touch, as Sari, a nurse working in home care, noted:

> Well, the primary purpose is to reduce the number of home visits. Of course, the use of technology also reduces the potential time when the nurse can touch the patient. But on the other hand, it again allows many old adults to live longer in their homes because they have a dispenser. (Sari, Finnish nurse)

Some robotics and other new technologies used in service work are becoming more socially interactive, providing also tactile simulations (Paterson, 2023). This is a form of social robotics, which is meant to help and encourage clients to interact with devices, replacing human interaction to some extent. Social robots are believed to bring comfort, especially to the lives of people suffering from loneliness, although

4.6 Work Automation, Cyborgs and Robotic Touch

they are not expected to completely replace human or animal companions. Examples of social robotics include animal-shaped robots such as the Paro seal, and small humanoid robots such the Nao robot with the Zora software, which has been especially used in the treatment of memory-impaired elderly patients. It is important to remember that the use of social robots in service work, education and nursing is still largely at the experimental stage, and we cannot know for sure whether they will play a major role in the future (Van Aerschot & Parviainen, 2020).

One of the few social robots whose use has become established in healthcare and utilises tactile stimulation is Paro, a device that looks like a seal pup. Paro can be held in one's lap, where it vibrates, moves and purrs when one strokes its fur. Many healthcare professionals we interviewed had positive experiences using Paro on memory units. 'Eila', an experienced nursing teacher who was the responsible teacher of geriatric nursing courses, for example, explained that the use of this robot was liberating because users did not need to worry about what the robot might think of them: unlike with human beings, there is no need to build an emotional bond with a robot. Paro could generate calming and empowering feelings and provide company in a similar way to dogs or cats. According to Eila, many older adults with dementia want to hold Paro because they need something they can pamper and hold in their arms. Certainly, many clients would prefer living animals, but electric animals can also be very attractive. It is important for residents not only to be touched but also to be agents who can touch others (e.g. pets or Paros). However, many nurses thought that technology should support the effectiveness of professionals' work tasks. Eila stressed during our interview that the use of technologies should not be a substitute for human interaction. This is why the use of Nao is more controversial among nurses than Paro.

The Nao robot (with Zora software installed) is a gesturing, talking device that resembles a human doll and is about half a metre tall. Although it is classified as a toy and entertainment device, suitable uses for it have been sought in both teaching and healthcare. Controlled from a laptop or similar device, Nao can be made to repeat sentences and enact sequences of motions. We have conducted experiments with it in nursing homes—for example, using it as a 'fitness instructor' for older adults (Parviainen et al., 2019). Its use proved to be time-consuming for the nursing home staff: while one person controlled the robot from the display, another had to repeat what it said, because many residents could not hear its speech. The findings of our experiments with Nao (Parviainen et al., 2019) confirmed the perceptions of the health professionals we interviewed. They thought that robots do not always make the professional's work tasks any easier; indeed, if anything, some robots are useless—or worse, even increase the professional's workload. A robot often needs extra efforts to support its function or, after all, the human professional must do its work. Further, some interviewees stated that robots were not always suitable to assist the elderly or the mentally ill, and they were sceptical that robots would provide sufficient benefits to make it worth introducing them into elderly care. Nonetheless, there is constant pressure to implement robots in nursing practices, since the robots have been developed by various companies in collaboration with healthcare professionals and organisations. 'Annika', a nursing teacher, doubted that robots would have any value for herself as companions in future:

Box 4.4 Three Approaches to Ethics in Care Robotics
The emergence of care robots has sparked ethical and social concerns over their potential effects on vulnerable groups such as children and older adults. Within this ethical debate we discern three different approaches to ethics, related to the researchers' different perspectives and disciplines. We call these approaches (1) the ethics of care robotics (i.e. advocates for philosophical ethics), (2) the ethical use of robotics in care (i.e. advocates for engineering care), and (3) robotics from the perspective of the ethics of caring (i.e. advocates for human care). While these approaches may intersect in many interdisciplinary studies—such as Sherry Turkle's (2012) book *Alone Together?*—researchers often limit their approach to ethics to perspectives from their own discipline. First, the ethics of care robotics is represented by professional philosophers (e.g. Vallor, 2016; van Wynsberghe, 2015). This approach is associated with specialist philosophical explorations (e.g. of ontological questions) and the application of ethical theories to robotics and technology. Second, the ethical use of robotics in care is mainly found in engineering science research, and it considers ethical issues from the viewpoint of technological innovations or management (e.g. Fosch-Villaronga & Albo-Canals, 2019; Yew, 2021). These scholars are interested in advancing the use of robotics in human care, for which they seek to develop appropriate ethical and legal criteria. Third, the ethics of caring is associated with research on human care and nursing science from the perspective of the humanities or social sciences (e.g. Stokes & Palmer, 2020; Van Aerschot & Parviainen, 2020; Wright, 2023). These researchers stress the principles of basic care, including safety, medication, communication, hydration, feeding, personal hygiene, dressing, rest and sleep, pain relief and dignity, among other things (Tronto, 1993). They also suggest that the most essential aspects of care—attentiveness, empathy, encountering the person and responding to their changing needs and situations—call for a human presence. Discussions of touch are mainly to be found in the ethics of caring approach. For instance, Bush (2001), Connor (2015), Connor and Howett (2009), and Stokes and Palmer (2020) suggest that a caring touch is one way to recognise and give dignity to the patient, bringing about comfort and security. Although care robots are expected to touch, lift and carry patients in future, many nursing researchers argue that robots cannot convey the same interpersonal affects through their touch as humans can—or at least, not without deception or delusion. Despite the differences among the three approaches, there is also some consensus among many researchers regarding ethics in care robotics: the right way to implement robotics in nursing is to use technologies in assistive roles (or as partners), not as substitutes for humans.

I find it a bit of a scary thought if I am thinking of myself as a memory-impaired person in a nursing home in the future. In the morning, a robot would come into the room to say 'good morning' when I wouldn't know where I was and who I was. So suddenly I would have that kind of robotic sound next to me. (Annika, Finnish nursing teacher)

Annika's fears resemble many nursing home residents' attitudes who were interviewed in our earlier project. The residents said that they would find it oppressive and scary if robots were to take care of them. However, many nurses thought it would be a good development if new technological applications, intelligent devices, lifting aids and wristband alarms were to be used in the care of the elderly. Nonetheless, some nurses were also concerned about the relative lack of attention to autonomy and self-sufficiency in discussions of assistive technologies. For example, is it ethically correct for a client to be required to wear a wristband? Wristbands can provide security for memory-impaired patients who live alone and receive home care a couple of times a day—for instance, the wristband can be used to check that the client is not going outside in freezing winter weather. On the other hand, the use of wristbands might lead to the reduction of home care visits, and the client's relatives may start to assume that the elderly person is fine living alone even if they have no opportunities to go outside or have face-to-face human contact. The danger is that old persons will become trapped alone in their homes, monitored by intelligent devices.

4.7 Material Touching: When Artefacts Touch You

> It is pitch black, and eerily quiet. I am floating in a foot of salt water, inside a light-proof, sound-proof tank. The air and the water are about the same temperature as my skin, and I realize I'm not sure where my body ends and my surroundings begin. I suddenly feel dizzy, and a wave of nausea washes over me. (DiBenedetto, 2016)

One of the most influential formulations developed in Merleau-Ponty's (1968) phenomenology concerns the touch of inanimate things, whether natural objects (e.g. trees) or human-made artefacts (e.g. tea cups). The main difference between human-human interaction and human-artefact interaction is the lack of reversibility: robots and other artefacts do not feel affective touch in the way that humans and animals do. Even though robots' sensors can be designed to respond as if they feel a touch, the fact remains that artefacts do not sense anything. Some people even prefer the 'passive' touch of objects because they find the social dimension of touch burdensome. Thus, despite our discussion in Sect. 4.6, the sensations and experiences produced by material objects and robot technologies may not be purely negative, and visions of a robotic future need not be entirely dystopian (Coghlan, 2021).

In the design of the environment, more and more attention has been paid to the pleasant sensory experiences that various artefacts can offer, especially in relation to the sense of touch. For example, schools have moved from rows of desks to beanbags and sitting balls, from blackboards to touch screens. Adults' touch memories of school may be associated with sharp-cornered, heavy wooden desks where the teacher told them to sit upright, quietly and still. Thus, technological changes in touch culture can apply to the learning environment, which in turn has a major influence on whether students consider the teaching to be meaningful and inspiring.

In addition, material devices can also relate directly to the pedagogical content of new teaching tools. For example, students can be taken on school trips to forests or museums, where they will get close to—and in the best-case scenario, touch—real historical, artistic or natural objects. Unlike with audio-visual materials on a screen, this material relationship is deeper and more diverse in terms of knowledge. Dreyfus's (2000) phenomenological approach to material artefacts can be useful here, especially if one looks at touch and haptics from an epistemic perspective. As Dreyfus (2000, p. 57) argues, 'what gives our sense of being in direct touch with reality is that we bring about changes in the world and get perceptual feedback concerning what we have done'. According to Dreyfus, we can only understand the world around us by exploring our environment through touch and bodily movement and receiving some kind of physical response and feedback from it.

Drawing on Merleau-Ponty's (1968) conceptualisation of the tactile, Erika Kerruish (2017) discusses the tactile sensations that material artefacts can provide to users. She considers that each tactile perception is embedded in an embodied imagination that includes memories, ideals, and cultural norms and values, among other things (Merleau-Ponty, 1989). Tactile meanings emerge from human embodied perception and the messy materialism of the device in which the discrete units of the digital are instantiated. Sensations provoked through touching are never completely precise or predictable. This comes close to Ihde's fourth formulation of technological mediation, that is, background relations (see Box 4.2). Ihde (1990) refers here to technologies such as refrigerators and air conditioners that provide pleasant material aid for us to live and work. In workplaces, background relations moderate various forms of touch between professionals and clients. For example, in the beautician's room, quiet soothing music, a soft sleeping pad and pleasant fragrances can help the client to fall asleep while the beautician cleanses and treats their skin. Another example is the tactilely stimulating learning environments we mentioned above. Such background relations can also include luxury wellness services, such as comfortable hotel beds that provide for the client's recreation or relaxation in the midst of a hectic life.

In floatation therapy, the experience of relaxation in specially made pods or tanks is generated by salt water that is the same temperature as one's skin.[1] The water pressure and temperature create the feeling that the body is effortlessly floating, defying gravity. While this floating eliminates the senses of touch, hearing, sight and smell, it simultaneously intensifies the feeling of the whole body, with some health benefits (Kjellgren & Westman, 2014). Skin and body weight provide the opportunity to feel like a whole body that is merging with the water. Floatation tanks are examples of technological devices as material actors that activate our bodies without being social

---

[1] The first tank was designed in 1954 by John C. Lilly, an American doctor and neuroscientist. He designed the tank in order to study the origins of consciousness by cutting off all external stimuli.

or claiming to expand our cognitive capacity. Such material technologies can also be liberating, because their human users do not need to be alert to any other sentient actors, providing an option to bypass cognitive stress.

The designers behind many digital applications have also sought to create or evoke feelings of touch, developing technical surfaces and materials to attract certain types of touch. The success of Apple's iPhone as the market leader in 2007 was based on its ability to deliver a pleasurable haptic experience: the swipe. With swiping, there is high overall consistency across haptics between the hand movement and the static visual information (i.e. images) on the surface. The feelings of pleasure caused by kinetic touch were subsequently exploited by many other devices. The Apple Watch can create vibrations that simulate the user's heartbeat, which can then be sent to other people as an intimate form of communication. Paro's combination of a furry surface and vibrations produced by sensors evokes a calming, relaxing form of pleasure in the user. Similarly, the Parihug, a stuffed animal especially designed for children, receives haptic hugs sent by loved ones who are far away. Such devices offer technological solutions to the yearning for human intimacy and touch.

In the future, touch-based technological solutions may lead to a new ecosystem of devices for lonely older adults, middle-aged people who need intimate partners and children whose parents no longer have time to hug them. Paradoxically, digital distance has created a market for technologies that simulate the touch and intimacy of others. While many people in the Western world find themselves deprived of touch, there are more and more novel technological solutions that provide sensory stimuli— for example, extended reality, which enables one to experience new worlds or add new facets to one's current reality.

4.8 Touch Deprivation in Digitised Working Environments?

> I don't think we should ever shake hands ever again, to be honest with you. Not only would it be good to prevent coronavirus disease, it probably would decrease instances of influenza dramatically in this country. (Fauci, interviewed by Linebaugh, 2020)

Experts such as Anthony Fauci have predicted that touch cultures will not recover from the COVID-19 pandemic, and that there will be permanent changes to the ways we touch each other in everyday life. Presumably, the ways in which professionals interact are also changing, and this development will be further accelerated by the transition to digital interactions. The pandemic accelerated a new global culture of remote working during 2020, when millions of white-collar employees, students and many others rapidly adjusted to working from home as their offices closed. Video conferencing replaced physical meetings and events. Business travel collapsed, and video conferencing across different time zones required people to extend their working hours into the late evening or bring them forwards to the early morning. Many parents had to work while simultaneously taking care of their young children or organising home schooling for them. Switching from one video conference to the next without a break while taking care of the children turned many home offices into chaotic environments. Nevertheless, in many jobs the worker's physical presence was still necessary, including hospital staff, supermarket assistants, refuse collectors and warehouse workers, who had to change their work habits and follow protective clothing protocols to prevent the new coronavirus from spreading.

Paradoxically, the pandemic also revealed the dimensions of physical presence and touch practices in different jobs and professions. Professions can be characterised in terms of the degree to which they require the physical presence or touch of co-workers or clients and the types of interaction required, whether outdoors or indoors. For instance, medical interventions for the treatment of acute cases require the physical presence of professionals and contact with the patient; transport work needs the driver's physical presence but allows them to maintain some physical distance from clients and artefacts. Work practices that involve higher levels of physical proximity and touch are likely to see greater transformations in the wake of the pandemic, because people may tend to remain cautious about physical touch even when there is no longer a risk of infection (Lund et al., 2021). In office work contexts, remote working and virtual meetings are likely to continue, albeit less intensely than during pandemic lockdown periods. Some customer interaction work, including front-line work in retail and banking, has accelerated the transition to e-commerce and other digital transactions. In the longer term, the shift to remote office working and the digitalisation of front-line services may lead to diminished customer-facing interactions, meaning fewer opportunities to cultivate forms of interaction based on touch.

The COVID-19 pandemic became a kind of global human experiment in which hundreds of millions of people spent months learning not to touch each other and to avoid being touched. It was the first time in millennia that such huge numbers of people had voluntarily refrained from fulfilling their inherent need to touch and be touched as part of everyday life in interaction with others.[2] While numerous studies have noted the alarming increase in mental health problems during the pandemic, some researchers have explored the role of touch—or more importantly, the lack of it—as yet another significant aspect of COVID-19. One reason for the low level of physical contact between people is that digital connectivity has become as ubiquitous as the air we breathe, as we mentioned at the beginning of this chapter. Retreating behind our digital shields and keeping our digital distance degrades our ability to engage in multisensory communication and encounter people as whole beings. In workplaces, people are shifting their personal communications to text messages and emails rather than talking by phone or meeting in person. New devices and applications are enthusiastically being developed, especially for traditionally touch-intensive basic services such as social care, healthcare and education.

Recent research findings suggest that a growing number of people are experiencing touch starvation due to the global COVID-19 pandemic (Brooke & Clark, 2020; Durkin et al., 2020; Golaya, 2021; Nist et al., 2020; Pierce, 2020). 'Touch starvation' refers to the desire for physical contact that humans and animals may experience after

---

[2] Of course, the COVID-19 pandemic is not the first pandemic that has sparked discussion about the importance of touch in human interaction (see Connor, 2015).

having little or no physical interaction with others over a period of time (Holler, 2002). For some individuals, this desire may feel similar to the desire for food when one is hungry. Touch starvation is also called 'touch depression', 'affection deprivation', 'touch hunger' or 'skin hunger'. It can lead to psychological complications, although there are also ways to help prevent it. Social distancing, lockdowns and other social restrictions to limit the spread of the virus prevented millions of people from interacting with and experiencing tactile contact with others. Numerous studies have shown that touch starvation can have various negative effects, including aggressive behaviours, speech and communication impairments, lowered self-esteem, and an increase in anxiety, depression, self-harm and eating disorders (Field, 2002; Golaya, 2021; Gupta & Schork, 1995; Turp, 2000).

While touch starvation can be understood as a psychological and individual state of mind, we want to stress that it is first and foremost a culturally and socially shaped situation. Touch starvation is often the result of cultural and social conditions characterised by touch deprivation. Some studies indicate that modern societies are developing into touch-deprived (Linden, 2015) or even touch-phobic cultures (Hertenstein et al., 2009). Touch deprivation may concern one or more groups in society. Old adults who live alone are one group at risk of touch deprivation, especially as home care is increasingly provided remotely. For instance, in the UK, half a million older people go for at least five or six days a week without seeing or speaking to anyone at all—and thus, without touching or being touched by another human (Age UK, 2018). However, older citizens are not the only people in this position; many young people are also at risk of exclusion from physical contact with and touch by other people. In Japan, *hikikomori* (引き篭もり) is a social withdrawal syndrome that occurs among teenagers and young adults, especially young males. Japan's Ministry of Labour, Welfare and Health has defined *hikikomori* as a person who is isolated from social relationships and the surrounding society for more than six months. A *hikikomori* does not go to school or work and has no close relationships outside the family; they mainly focus on computers and gaming. Estimates suggest that half a million young Japanese people have become social recluses, as have more than half a million middle-aged individuals. Therefore, in both Western and Eastern high-tech societies, touch deprivation has not only been caused by the COVID-19 pandemic but is also related to cultural conditions resulting from much longer-term developments in digital technologies and lifestyles.

In his book *The Senses of Touch: Haptics, Affects and Technologies*, Paterson (2007) discusses how the spatially proximate sense of touch can be digitised and experienced over distance, a phenomenon he calls 'mediated touch' or 'a sense of presence of a distant other' (Haans & Ijsselsteijn, 2006, p. 153). He is interested in how the sense of presence at a distance is enhanced through haptic technologies. While technology has facilitated long-distance interactions in the auditory and visual realms, the development of applications for long-distance interpersonal touch is still in its infancy (Haans & Ijsselsteijn, 2006). After twenty years of hope and hype, this telepresence touch technology is just starting to appear in consumer electronics. By blending the real and virtual worlds, extended reality (augmented reality, virtual reality and mixed reality) creates an immersive experience that is used not only for entertainment but also as a working tool—for example, to teach history in schools or to train pilots in the military. Although these devices provide opportunities to discover new (imaginary) worlds through haptic gloves, they also keep people physically distant from the world and people around them. It is almost ironic that these haptic technologies provide restrictive proxies for touch perception. They create the illusion that one is touching something, but they prevent one from experiencing the feeling of really touching anything.

Paterson (2007) is primarily interested in conveying online haptic experiences between two people—online handshakes, so to speak. As engineers who work with long-distance interpersonal haptics understand, the haptic system comprises more than the skin's surface. If one wishes to recreate the 'authentic' haptic feel of touching somebody, it must include features such as the proper temperature, pressure, vibration and texture on the skin, combined with gestures. What is significant here is the user (toucher)-oriented intention to engender the right 'feel'. While the hope of generating the sensory and spatial effects of touch at a distance has posed many engineering challenges, perhaps the main problem is that consumers have simply not adopted the technology. The mimetic nature of a haptic experience recreated through digital means is unambiguously illusory—a phantom-like presence (Paterson, 2007). The obstacle to a wider consumer take-up of virtual touch devices may be that consumers are unwilling to adopt a new language of haptic sensation while using such devices. Although tactile sensory properties are mimicked, modelled, experimented with and reproduced through the interaction between hardware and software, consumers do not find the results sufficiently attractive to spend money on. Thus, haptic online technologies are not necessarily the best solution for global problems related to touch deprivation.

In conclusion, Table 4.1 brings together the key concepts discussed in this chapter to describe the roles played by touch when various technologies and tools are used in service work. We have described how the mechanical tools, instruments and digital technologies used by professionals both enable and prevent physical contact with clients. Devices, tools and robotics expand the capabilities of the working body, but at the same time they shape our physiology, living body and habitus. Professionals must learn to manage all of the communication problems, interpersonal tensions and affects that the touch of technologies and materials brings to service interactions.

4.9 Thematic Learning Tasks

4.9.1 Reflection Activities

1. Think about a normal working day in your own job or, alternatively, for example, an internship related to your future profession. Consider the following questions:
   - What kind of technology-mediated interaction is part of your job? Try to list all the devices, instruments, tools, etc. that you use during the day to interact with the client.

4.9 Thematic Learning Tasks

Table 4.1 Summary of key concepts related to technology-mediated touch

Key concept	Meaning	Impact on nature of touch	Examples
Automation	Enhancements to work productivity through a wide range of technologies that reduce human cognitive and physical interventions in work processes	Has negative impacts on touching when work becomes routine and touching has no place, and positive impacts when automation offers the opportunity to create tactile interactions with the client	Patient enrolment machines, robotic drug delivery
Bodily extensions	Enhancements of sensorimotor, visual and hearing capabilities in particular	Enables professionals to touch clients with instruments or at a distance through visual-haptic technologies	Surgical robots, stethoscopes
Cyborgs	A combination of the cybernetic and the organic, with both organic and biomechatronic body parts	Enhances human biological capabilities, thereby indirectly impacting on touching	Hearing implants, exoskeletons
Digital distance	Digital barriers between people who are present to each other physically but whose attention is focused on digital content rather than on personal interaction	Has a negative influence on interacting with and touching the other person	Typing up patient notes while talking to the patient
Digital proxemics	How social space with other people is perceived and acted upon in malleable virtual environments and digital spaces	Has both negative and positive impacts on touching	Echo chambers as social media bubbles
Digitalisation	Increased adoption of digital technologies to revise extant organisational processes and work practices	Reduces (but does not eliminate) the use of physical contact in client interactions, thereby shaping forms of touching	Fostering of the primacy of technology over humans
Gathering-around technologies	Social, personal or intimate zones between people when the use of technologies connects and activates people to work or play together	Promotes and intensifies interactions in face-to-face encounters	Reading and looking at pictures on a tablet with a nursery schoolchild
Material touch	Pleasant or unpleasant tactile experiences provided by artefacts, technologies and natural materials	Can be desirable and relaxing because the 'passivity' of material touch removes the social burden of touching	Floatation tanks, touch screens
Social robotics	Autonomous or semi-autonomous human- or animal-like machines that interact with humans and are programmed to follow certain rules of social behaviour	Provides human-like or animal-like gestures and touch interactions with humans	Humanoid robots, animal-shaped robots, hugging robots

(continued)

Table 4.1 (continued)

Key concept	Meaning	Impact on nature of touch	Examples
Technology-mediated touch	Research approach and umbrella concept covering various forms of interaction in which technological devices and tools modify and shape the touch experience between the professional and the client	Entails numerous forms of touching with technologies and tools in client interactions	Gathering-around technologies, touching with and through technologies, triadic touch, material touch
Touch deprivation	A result of cultural and social conditions where touching is avoided for health, technological or other reasons	Significantly hinders the cultivation and development of touch culture	Social distancing, lockdowns and social restrictions to limit the spread of COVID-19
Touching with and through technologies	Technologies and tools professionals use that form intelligent extensions of and reshape their bodies and perceptions while helping them to develop affective relations with clients	Entails numerous forms of touching in interactions	A barber using scissors and a comb simultaneously while cutting the client's hair
Triadic touch	Technologies that operate as actors between professional and client, thereby potentially forming organisational-level systems that influence touch in interactive work	Endows technologies with their own kinds of touch, and requires the professional to modify the experience of technological touch through speech or other activities if the client feels uncomfortable	Inserting a cannula

- How much of your working day consists of technology-mediated touch and digital interaction with the client compared to face-to-face interaction?
- Do you find the technology-mediated interaction pleasant or does it cause you anxiety or stress?

2. Think about the organisation where you work and/or where you are going to work after your studies:
   - What kind of culture prevails there in terms of digitalisation and technologies?
   - Is there an attempt to steer customer interaction more and more in a technology-mediated direction, or is the importance of face-to-face contact emphasised?
   - In respect of technology use, to what extent can the organisation and your colleagues support or hinder the development of work practices in which physical touch is taken into account?

3. Put yourself in the client's shoes and think about how they perceive your interaction with them in and through various technologies:
   - Does the use of devices take up too much of your time in your work? How could you focus better on the client's needs?
   - How can you better negotiate the client's potential fears or any unpleasant feelings produced by the technologies you use?
   - What kind of capabilities do you have for managing communication problems, interpersonal tensions and the affects that the touch of technologies and materials brings to the service interaction?
4. Think about what new insights and learnings this chapter has awakened in you:
   - What kind of skills and competences do you already hold in terms of technology-mediated touch in interactive client work, that you had not previously recognised?
   - What weaknesses or limitations have you found in your technology-mediated touch that you could work further to overcome?
   - What kind of support would you need and from whom for this development?

4.9.2 Fieldwork

Digitisation has had a significant impact on the work of many different professionals. However, little is known so far about how digitalisation affects tactile interaction in the service sector. You can advance this knowledge by conducting a little field research on this topic. Think of someone in your close circle (friends, relatives) who has a relatively long work history, say 10–20 years, in the service sector (health care, education, fitness, etc). Ask this person if you could interview them about the impact of digitalisation in how different technologies are changing how they interact with clients. Tell them that the interview is related to your studies and this textbook. You can take notes about the interview or ask their consent to record the interview. Focus on touching and physical contact when using technologies. You can ask them, for example:

- Has digitalisation reduced or increased touch interaction in the past ten years?
- What new technologies have been developed that facilitate or hinder the interaction between a professional and a client?
- Has the COVID-19 pandemic changed touch practices in their work environment?

4.9.3 Case Study

Read the following story and consider how technology-mediated touch shapes the interaction between a doctor and a patient by answering the questions below.

Anna works as a doctor in a health centre. Arriving at her workplace, her first task is to open the computer to see who her first patient is. She reads a short description of the patient's symptoms in the database and checks whether they have already registered via the registration machine in the lobby. The patient appears to be waiting in the lobby, with a numbered ticket from the machine in his hand. Anna calls them in by pressing her room number on the notice board, and the patient enters. Anna greets the patient by nodding, but says she does not shake his hand in line with new post-pandemic guidance. She asks the patient to sit down and kindly asks what is bothering him. The patient tells her he has had a pressing pain in his ear for several days. Anna nods and says that she will wash her hands before examining the patient's ear more closely. She takes an otoscope light to examine the patient's ear. Positioning herself sideways to the patient, she gently touches the patient's shoulder, while she explains what she is going to do. She carefully pulls the patient's earlobe up and back so that the ear canal straightens and the eardrum is better visible. She detects inflammation in the eardrum. Anna tells the patient how the ear should be treated. She will rinse the ear clean with a saline solution and then drip a combination antibiotic/cortisone medicine into the ear. The patient nods as a sign of agreement. Anna performs the procedure and writes the patient's antibiotics and painkillers on an electronic prescription. The patient is relieved, although the ear is still sore. He thanks Anna and leaves the room. Anna turns to the computer and dictates to the machine her diagnosis, the procedures performed and the medications prescribed. The patient can check his own information in the database. When going to the pharmacy, the patient can get the medicines by showing his identity card. Consider the following questions:

- In what ways does digitalisation frame and guide the interaction between doctor and patient?
- Describe how touching with and through technologies appears in this encounter.
- How do you characterise triadic touch in this encounter?

References

Age UK. (2018). *Later life in the United Kingdom*. Retrieved October 16, 2018, from https://www.ageuk.org.uk/globalassets/age-uk/documents/reports-and-publications/later_life_uk_factsheet.pdf

Anderson, J., & Ranie, L. (2018). *Stories from experts about the impact of digital life* (pp. 1–6). Pew Research Center. https://www.pewresearch.org/internet/2018/07/03/stories-from-experts-about-the-impact-of-digital-life/

Arcega, J., Autman, I., De Guzman, B., et al. (2020). The human touch is modern technology decreasing the value of humanity in patient care? *Critical Care Nursing Quarterly, 43*(3), 294–302.

Baker, C. C. (2019). *New directions in mobile media and performance*. Routledge.

Bali, J., Garg, R., & Bali, R. (2019). Artificial intelligence (AI) in healthcare and biomedical research: Why a strong computational/AI bioethics framework is required? *Indian Journal of Ophthalmology, 67*(1), 3. https://doi.org/10.4103/ijo.ijo_1292_18

Barron Rodriguez, M. R., Cobo Romani, J. C., Munoz-Najar, A., & Sanchez Ciarrusta, I. A. (2022). *Remote learning during the global school lockdown: Multi-country lessons*. World Bank Group. http://documents.worldbank.org/curated/en/668741627975171644/Remote-Learning-During-the-Global-School-Lockdown-Multi-Country-Lessons

References

Bondanini, G., Giorgi, G., Ariza-Montes, A., Vega-Muñoz, A., & Andreucci-Annunziata, P. (2020). Technostress dark side of technology in the workplace: A scientometric analysis. *International Journal of Environmental Research and Public Health, 17*(21), 8013. https://doi.org/10.3390/ijerph17218013

Bourdieu, P. (1990). *The logic of practice* (R. Nice, Trans.). Stanford University Press.

Bourdieu, P., & Wacquant, L. J. D. (1992). *An invitation to reflexive sociology*. University of Chicago Press.

Brod, C. (1984). *Technostress: The human cost of the computer revolution*. Addison-Wesley Publishing Company.

Brooke, J., & Clark, M. (2020). Older people's early experience of household isolation and social distancing during COVID-19. *Journal of Clinical Nursing, 29*, 4387–4402.

Bush, E. (2001). The use of human touch to improve the well-being of older adults: A holistic nursing intervention. *Journal of Holistic Nursing, 19*(3), 256–270.

Coghlan, S. (2021). Robots and the possibility of humanistic care. *International Journal of Social Robotics*. https://doi.org/10.1007/s12369-021-00804-7

Connor, A. (2015). Touch in the age of Ebola. *Nursing Outlook, 63*(1), 25–26. https://doi.org/10.1016/j.outlook.2014.11.016

Connor, A., & Howett, M. (2009). A conceptual model of intentional comfort touch. *Journal of Holistic Nursing, 27*(2), 127–135. https://doi.org/10.1177/0898010109333337

Crossley, N. (2007). Researching embodiment by way of 'body techniques'. *The Sociological Review, 55*(1 Suppl), 80–94. https://doi.org/10.1111/j.1467-954X.2007.00694.x

De Saint Laurent, C. (2018). In defence of machine learning: Debunking the myths of artificial intelligence. *Europe's Journal of Psychology, 14*(4), 734.

Dean, S., Lewis, J., & Ferguson, C. (2017). Editorial: Is technology responsible for nurses losing touch? *Journal of Clinical Nursing, 26*(5–6), 583–585. https://doi.org/10.1111/jocn.13470

DiBenedetto, C. (2016). The crazy thing that happened when I tried floating in a soundproof, lightproof tank. *Health*, April 28, 2016. https://www.health.com/mind-body/floatation-therapy

Dragano, N., & Lunau, T. (2020). Technostress at work and mental health: Concepts and research results. *Current Opinion in Psychiatry, 33*(4), 407–413. https://doi.org/10.1097/YCO.0000000000000613

Dreyfus, H. L. (1992). *What computers still can't do: A critique of artificial reason*. MIT Press.

Dreyfus, H. L. (2000). Telepistemology: Descartes' last stand. In K. Goldberg (Ed.), *The Robot in the garden: Telerobotics and telepistemology in the age of the Internet* (pp. 48–63). MIT Press.

Durkin, J., Jackson, D., & Usher, K. (2020). Touch in times of COVID-19: Touch hunger hurts. *Journal of Clinical Nursing, 30*, e4–e5.

Field, T. (2002). Infants' need for touch. *Human Development, 45*, 100–103.

Fosch-Villaronga, E., & Albo-Canals, J. (2019). "I'll take care of you", said the robot. *Paladyn, Journal of Behavioral Robotics, 10*, 77–93.

Frey, C. B., & Osborne, M. A. (2017). The future of employment: How susceptible are jobs to computerisation? *Technological Forecasting and Social Change, 114*, 254–280.

Golaya, S. (2021). Touch-hunger: An unexplored consequence of the COVID-19 pandemic. *Indian Journal of Psychological Medicine, 43*(4), 362–363. https://doi.org/10.1177/02537176211014469

Gupta, M. A., & Schork, N. J. (1995). Touch deprivation has an adverse effect on body image: Some preliminary observations. *The International Journal of Eating Disorders, 17*, 185–189.

Haans, A., & Ijsselsteijn, W. (2006). Mediated social touch: A review of current research and future directions. *Virtual Reality, 9*, 149–159.

Haddad, A., Doherty, R., & Purtilo, R. (2019). Respectful communication in an information age. In W. B. Saunders (Ed.), *Health professional and patient interaction* (9th ed., pp. 141–165). Elsevier. https://doi.org/10.1016/B978-0-323-53362-1.00010-4

Hall, E. T. (1963). A system for the notation of proxemic behavior. *American Anthropologist, 65*(5), 1003–1026.

Haraway, D. (1985). A manifesto for cyborgs: Science, technology, and socialist feminism in the 1980s. *Socialist Review, 80*, 65–108.

Haraway, D. (1997). *Modest_witness@second_millennium.femaleman_meets_oncomouse*. Routledge.
Haraway, D. (2003). *The companion species manifesto: Dogs, people, and significant otherness*. Prickly Paradigm Press.
Harbers, H. (2005). Introduction: Co-production, agency, and normativity. In H. Harbers (Ed.), *Inside the politics of technology: Agency and normativity in the co-production of technology and society* (pp. 9–25). Amsterdam University Press.
Hayles, N. K. (1999). *How we became posthuman: Virtual bodies in cybernetics, literature, and informatics*. Chicago University Press.
Hertenstein, M. J., Holmes, R., Keltner, D., & McCullough, M. (2009). The communication of emotion via touch. *Emotion, 9*(4), 566–573.
Holler, L. (2002). *Erotic morality: The role of touch in moral agency*. Rutgers University Press.
HUS (The Hospital District of Helsinki and Uusimaa). (2021). Uusi Da Vinci Xi -leikkausrobotti vahvistaa HUSin roolia robottikirurgian kehittäjänä Euroopassa [The new Da Vinci Xi surgical robot strengthens HUS's role as a developer of robotic surgery in Europe]. Press release, November 10, 2021. https://www.hus.fi/ajankohtaista/uusi-da-vinci-xi-leikkausrobotti-vahvistaa-husin-roolia-robottikirurgian-kehittajana
Ihde, D. (1979). *Technics and praxis: A philosophy of technology*. Boston series in the philosophy of science. Reidel Press.
Ihde, D. (1990). *Technology and the lifeworld: From garden to earth*. Indiana University Press.
Ihde, D. (2001). *Bodies in technology*. University of Minnesota.
Kerruish, E. (2017). Affective touch in social robots. *Transformations, 29*, 116–135.
Kjellgren, A., & Westman, J. (2014). Beneficial effects of treatment with sensory isolation in flotation-tank as a preventive health-care intervention – A randomized controlled pilot trial. *BMC Complementary and Alternative Medicine, 14*, 417. https://doi.org/10.1186/1472-6882-14-417
Kraus, S., Schiavone, F., Pluzhnikova, A., & Invernizzi, A. C. (2021). Digital transformation in healthcare: Analyzing the current state-of-research. *Journal of Business Research, 123*, 557–567.
Kurki, E. (2022). Huoltajat ilmoittavat kouluun, ettei lapsen tarvitse lukea kirjoja, koska näin on kotona sovittu – Opettajat avautuvat, millaisilla asioilla vanhemmat piinaavat [Parents inform the school that the child does not need to read books, because this is what has been agreed at home – Teachers open up about what kinds of things parents torment them]. *Helsingin Sanomat*, August 21, 2022. https://www.hs.fi/kotimaa/art-2000009001096.html
Latour, B. (1993). *We have never been modern*. Harvard University Press.
Law, J., & Singleton, V. (2013). ANT and politics: Working in and on the world. *Qualitative Sociology, 36*, 485–502. https://doi.org/10.1007/s11133-013-9263-7
Linden, D. (2015). *Touch: The science of hand, heart and mind*. Penguin Books.
Linebaugh, K. (2020). Dr. Anthony Fauci on how life returns to normal. WSJ Podcast, July 4, 2020. https://www.wsj.com/podcasts/the-journal/dr-anthony-fauci-on-how-life-returns-to-normal/d5754969-7027-431e-89fa-e12788ed9879
Lund, S., Madgavkar, A., Manyika, J., et al. (2021). *The postpandemic economy: The future of work after COVID-19*. McKinsey Global Institute. https://www.mckinsey.com/~/media/mckinsey/featured%20insights/future%20of%20organizations/the%20future%20of%20work%20after%20covid%2019/the-future-of-work-after-covid-19-report-vf.pdf
Lupton, D. (2013). Quantifying the body: Monitoring and measuring health in the age of mHealth technologies. *Critical Public Health, 23*(4), 393–403. https://doi.org/10.1080/09581596.2013.794931
McArthur, J. A. (2016). *Digital proxemics. How technology shapes the ways we move*. Peter Lang.
Merleau-Ponty, M. (1968). *The visible and the invisible*. Followed by working notes, ed. C. Lefort (A. Lingis, Trans.). Northwestern University Press.
Merleau-Ponty, M. (1989). *The phenomenology of perception* (C. Smith, Trans.). Routledge. (Original work published 1945).

References

Müller, M., & Schur, C. (2016). Assemblage thinking and actor-network theory: Conjunctions, disjunctions, cross-fertilisations. *Transactions of the Institute of British Geographers*. https://doi.org/10.1111/tran.12117

Nguyen, C. T. (2022). How twitter gamifies communication. In J. Lackey (Ed.), *Applied epistemology* (pp. 410–436). Oxford University Press.

Nist, M. D., Harrison, T. M., Tate, J., Robinson, A., Balas, M., & Pickler, R. H. (2020). Losing touch. *Nursing Inquiry, 27*, e12368.

Palumbo, R. (2021). Does digitizing involve desensitizing? Strategic insights into the side effects of workplace digitization. *Public Management Review, 24*(7), 975–1000. https://doi.org/10.1080/14719037.2021.1877796

Palumbo, R., & Cavallone, M. (2022). Is work digitalization without risk? Unveiling the psychosocial hazards of digitalization in the education and healthcare workplace. *Technology Analysis & Strategic Management*. https://doi.org/10.1080/09537325.2022.2075338

Parviainen, J., & Pirhonen, J. (2017). Vulnerable bodies in human-robot interaction: Embodiment as ethical issue in robot care for the elderly. *Transformation, 29*, 104–115. http://www.transformationsjournal.org/wp-content/uploads/2017/02/Transformations29_Parviainen-Pirhonen.pdf

Parviainen, J., & Rantala, J. (2021). Chatbot breakthrough in the 2020s? An ethical reflection on the trend of automated consultations in health care. *Medicine, Health Care and Philosophy, 25*(1), 61–71. https://doi.org/10.1007/s11019-021-10049-w

Parviainen, J., Van Aerschot, L., Särkikoski, T., et al. (2019). Motions with emotions? A phenomenological approach to understand the simulated aliveness of a robot body. *Techné: Research in Philosophy and Technology, 23*(3), 318–341. https://doi.org/10.5840/techne20191126106

Paterson, M. (2007). *The senses of touch: Haptics, affects and technologies*. Taylor & Francis Group.

Paterson, M. (2023). Social robots and the futures of affective touch. *The Senses and Society*. https://doi.org/10.1080/17458927.2023.2179231

Piaget, J. (1970). *The principles of genetic epistemology*. Routledge & Kegan Paul.

Pierce, S. (2020). Touch starvation is a consequence of COVID-19's physical distancing. TMC, 15 May, 2020. https://www.tmc.edu/news/2020/05/touch-starvation/

Pykett, J., & Paterson, M. (2022). Stressing the 'body electric': History and psychology of the techno-ecologies of work stress. *History of the Human Sciences, 35*(5), 185–212.

Rajamanickam, L., Raiyan, F., & Hamza, M. (2022). Impact of intelligent automation and digitalization on human labour. *International Journal of Mechanical Engineering, 7*(1), 1345–1349.

Scott, D., & Purves, I. N. (1996). Triadic relationship between doctor, computer and patient. *Interacting with Computers, 8*(4), 347363. https://doi.org/10.1016/S0953-5438(97)83778-2

Sheets-Johnstone, M. (1999). *The primacy of movement*. John Benjamins.

Stokes, F., & Palmer, A. (2020). Artificial intelligence and robotics in nursing: Ethics of caring as a guide to dividing tasks between AI and humans. *Nursing Philosophy*. https://doi.org/10.1111/nup.12306

Thrift, N. (2000). Afterwords. *Environment and Planning D*. https://doi.org/10.1068/d214t

Tronto, J. C. (1993). *Moral boundaries: A political argument for an ethic of care*. Psychology Press.

Turkle, S. (2012). *Alone together? Why we expect more from technology and less from each other?* Basic Books.

Turp, M. (2000). Touch, enjoyment and health: In adult life. *European Journal of Psychotherapy and Counselling, 3*, 33–46.

Vallor, S. (2016). *Technology and the virtues: A philosophical guide to a future worth wanting*. Oxford University Press.

Van Aerschot, L., & Parviainen, J. (2020). Robots responding to care needs? A multitasking care robot pursued for 25 years, available products offer simple entertainment and instrumental assistance. *Ethics and Information Technology, 22*, 247–256. https://doi.org/10.1007/s10676-020-09536-0

van Wynsberghe, A. (2015). *Healthcare robots: Ethics, design and implementation*. Routledge.

Wajcman, J. (2004). *TechnoFeminism*. Polity Press.

Wright, J. A. (2023). *Robots won't save Japan. An ethnography of eldercare automation*. ILR Press.
Yew, G. C. K. (2021). Trust in and ethical design of carebots: The case for ethics of care. *International Journal of Social Robotics, 13*, 629–645. https://doi.org/10.1007/s12369-020-00653-w

Further Reading

de Vaujany, F. X., Adrot, A., Boxenbaum, E., & Leca, B. (2019). *Materiality in institutions: Spaces, embodiment and technology in management and organization*. Palgrave.
Dourish, P. (2001). *Where the action is: The foundations of embodied interaction*. MIT Press.
Küpers, W. (2014). *Phenomenology of the embodied organization: The contribution of Merleau-Ponty for organizational studies and practice*. Palgrave.
Lupton, D. (2018). *Digital healthcare. Critical and cross-disciplinary perspectives*. Routledge.
McDowell, L. (2011). *Working bodies: Interactive service employment and workplace identities*. Wiley.
Paulsen, K. (2017). *Here/there: Telepresence, touch, and art at the interface*. MIT Press.
Suchman, L. A. (2007). *Human–machine reconfigurations: Plans and situated action*. Cambridge University Press.
White, M. (2022). *Touch screen theory: Digital devices and feelings*. MIT Press.

The Ethics of Professional Touch 5

Abstract

This chapter introduces new principles of professional ethics for touch-based client work by drawing on the philosophy of ethics and research on touch and affects. Our motivation for doing this is the observation that many professionals struggle with dilemmas regarding the types of touch that are ethically appropriate in interactions with clients. Touch cultures have changed due to digitalisation, the demand for economic efficiency and the reduction of resources, #Metoo movement and the effects of COVID-19. We formulate an embodied ethics to provide principles regarding how professionals work with touching ethically sustainable ways, while taking account of the many factors that can limit touch interactions. The essence of touching is that one person can never touch another without being touched themselves. This reciprocity of touch has effects on professionals' work with clients. Therefore, it is important to consider rewarding feelings and the moral distress that touch can cause to professionals.

Introduction

In this chapter, we introduce new principles of professional ethics for touch-based client work by drawing on the philosophy of ethics and research on touch and affects. Our motivation for doing this is the observation that many professionals struggle with dilemmas regarding the types of touch that are ethically appropriate in interactions with clients. The culture of client work has changed due to digitalisation, the demand for economic efficiency and the reduction of resources, as well as the #Metoo movement and the effects of COVID-19. We formulate an embodied ethics to provide principles regarding how professionals can be present to, approach or behave towards clients in fair and ethically sustainable ways, while taking account of the many factors that can limit touch interactions. This ethics considers the client's needs, but above all, it rests on universal human rights, legal guidelines and professional well-being. The essence of touching is that one person can never touch another without being touched themselves. This reciprocity of touch has effects on professionals' work with clients, sometimes in unpredictable ways. Therefore, it is also important to consider the moral distress that touch can cause to professionals. Individual professionals can develop their own touch skills, and organisations' working practices can be enhanced in touch-sensitive ways.

Learning Objectives
In this chapter, you will familiarise yourself with the theory and principles of the ethics of professional touch, as well as the regulations, international recommendations and professional knowledge that justify it. After this you can

- identify the fundamental concepts and key issues of the ethics of touch
- discuss and analyse your own way of touching in relation to the client's needs, your organisation's touch culture and professional knowledge gained by education
- identify and analyse ethical dimensions and potential problem situations in touch interaction with the client
- describe what kind of beneficial features can be associated with the use of touch in client work

5.1 Touching as an Ethical Dilemma for Professionals

> I've felt guilty for sitting on the floor and doing what I really ought to do, what I have been trained for, where the core of this all is. And then the door opens, someone enters the room, and I feel as if someone is pointing an accusing finger at me because it looks like I am being lazy. Like I am just sitting there. 'Hey, please go and help another group!' Of course we must help other groups, but could the others also calm down and sit on the floor? (Raisa, Finnish early childhood educator, quoted in Puroila et al., 2018, p. 25)

This early childhood educator sat on the floor and held a child in her arms, a basic task in the education of children. At the same time, she also identified factors that threatened her performance of that task. Her insights into her basic task as a professional focused on the child's needs, the professional activity that would support the child's balanced growth and development, and her own professional ethical obligation to act accordingly. As she sat on the floor, perhaps she also wondered whether to prolong this close, sensitive moment with the child, even though she was simultaneously expected to obey the demands of her work community and her employer. This situation is a typical example of the messy ethical dilemmas (see also Bynum et al., 2014; Haahr et al., 2020; Hansson & Fröding, 2021; Hännikäinen, 2018; Karlsson et al., 2013; Puroila & Haho, 2017; Sipman et al., 2019) that arise when professionals have to navigate through the landscape of knowledge, rights, values, obligations, perceptions, attitudes, volitions, expectations and real life.

Today, professionals increasingly need sensitive skills of observation and presence if they are to perceive the ethical factors at play in their work. They often find themselves in situations where they must weigh their own conceptions of good and right against those of their environment, organisation, clients or colleagues. Clients and their family members, employers, and many others expect professionals to distinguish between right and wrong alternatives and make decisions in a professional way, altruistically and fairly. Professional decision-making and actions become especially important in ethical dilemmas that require choices about values. Regarding the ethics of touch, we call this type of prudence 'value awareness'. We will concretise this idea in relation to Martin Buber's (1993) philosophy of 'I and Thou', which offers an interesting framework for insights into how professionals make themselves present to the client, and how they invite the client to interact: the professional responds to the needs of the other through a touch that essentially respects the other person.

When it comes to the ethics of touch, professionals are forced to struggle with dilemmas regarding touch that is ethically appropriate and touch that should be considered wrong, bad or harmful. Professionals have become more and more aware of the factors that threaten their encounters with clients, such as the increasingly fast pace of client work, the effects of digitalisation on the reduction of client contact, or failures in efficiency. At the same time, the COVID-19 pandemic, the #Metoo movement and Black Lives Matter (BLM) protests have put the ethics of touch in a new spotlight, revealing that people have different views regarding the kinds of touch that may be vital, ethically justified, disturbing or abusive. For this reason, it is important for professionals to deeply understand the ethical principles behind their activities and to draw on different ethical approaches to justify and resolve their dilemmas. Therefore, we will now take a closer look at the normative guidelines and ethical principles behind professional touch.

5.2 Normative Ethics and Touch

Professional ethics as a form of applied ethics frequently includes rules or guidelines regarding how to apply normative ethics to practical problems. Thus, professional ethics is usually normative, and it aims to find the best possible answers to moral issues, although the practical issues involved in professional work are often so complicated that simple answers are not available. Normative ethics is concerned with the criteria we can use to distinguish moral right from wrong, or bad touches from good. Normative ethics includes the formulation of moral rules that are intended to have direct effects on people's actions, institutions and lifestyles.

In its simplest form, professional normative ethics consists of general and universal guidelines and codes. Various occupational groups have aligned themselves with national and international recommendations, regulations, standards, legislation and other common agreements or ethical codes to guide their client work. International recommendations differ little from each other within occupations, although there are minor differences in practical applications and the interpretations of main principles. For example, the World Health Organization's *Code of ethics and professional conduct* (WHO, 2022) considers social welfare and healthcare professionals to be bound by five values: integrity, accountability, independence and impartiality, respect, and professional commitment. The ethical code of the *World Medical Association* (WMA, 2022) and the *International code of ethics for nurses* (ICN, 2022) belong to the field of applied ethics and offer norms for practitioners in different specialist domains. In the field of education, ethical codes adhere to values that are roughly similar to those found in the social welfare and health sectors: respect for human dignity, truthfulness, solidarity and equality. Furthermore, the goal of teachers' ethics, according to the *International code of ethics for educators* (ICOEE, 2022), is to support and promote peace, sustainable development, social and economic stability, and global progress centred on human dignity.

In addition to such ethical codes, professionals need more specific ethical knowledge to be able to apply the codes in practice. Thomas Beauchamp and James Childress's (1985/2013) formulation of four principles—autonomy, non-maleficence, beneficence and justice—is one of the most widely used ethical frameworks and offers a broad consideration of professional ethics. Although Beauchamp and Childress provide universal principles, their everyday practical application often requires further ethical reflection. When it comes to questions of appropriate and inappropriate touch in client-professional interactions, Beauchamp and Childress' (1985/2013) approach requires us to interpret their formulations at the practical level, since they do not provide detailed guidance for real-life situations (see Box 5.1). For this reason, ethical rules or principles can easily remain abstract, especially when ethical practices are implemented mechanically in professional work. Typically, in practical work, professionals must make prompt decisions about their touch practices based on their own intuition and judgement.

However, it would be wrong to claim that experts do not need normative guidelines regarding how to use touch in their work. In fact, professionals frequently adhere to specific normative theories—often without being aware of what those theories are or what philosophical background they come from. To further understand how touching is related to traditional normative theories of ethics, we have formulated some ethical questions about touch and clarified how they align with well-known ethical theories (Table 5.1). We have formulated the questions to indicate how professionals usually justify their own tactile interactions (or lack of interaction) with their clients. Professional normative ethics deals with questions of touching in terms of rights, responsibilities, virtues, equality and willingness. Through these questions, professionals can identify the different normative ethical approaches that lie behind their own perceptions, actions and beliefs.

Classical theories of normative ethics provide criteria for morally right or wrong practices, the kind of person we should be and what we should strive for. Consequentialism (or teleological ethics) is target-oriented: the value of an act is determined by the consequences to which it leads. Consequentialists consider the beneficial or negative feelings a touch can produce in the client. The major tendency within consequentialism is utilitarianism, where the principle is to secure the greatest possible good for the greatest possible number of people. A utilitarian will ask how their touch will benefit their clients. Hedonist utilitarians, on the other hand, ask what kind of interaction will provide professionals themselves or the client as

> **Box 5.1 Touching from the Perspective of Beauchamp and Childress' Bioethical Principles**
>
> Beauchamp and Childress' (1985/2013) biomedical ethics describes four moral principles: autonomy, non-maleficence, beneficence and justice. The first principle, respect for autonomy, involves taking account of the client's individual opinions, expectations or needs during every encounter, unless they are detrimental to others. The principle of non-maleficence—'do no harm'—means that any unnecessary, harmful or unjustified action or treatment should be avoided, because all medicines and treatments always entail risks. Beneficence refers to acts of kindness, charity and altruism in the sense that a beneficent person does more than the bare minimum. The justice principle in Beauchamp and Childress' bioethics refers to the fair distribution of resources, which in healthcare contexts are often limited.
>
> Beauchamp and Childress (1985/2013) say little about how we should interpret autonomy, non-maleficence, beneficence and justice when we are considering appropriate and inappropriate touch in client—professional interactions. It is conceivable that touch in these encounters should encompass the client's humane and individual treatment, as well as tolerance for and consideration of the client's individual values, skills and resources. Applying Beauchamp and Childress' four core concepts to touch, we propose the following interpretations:
>
> **Autonomy** in professional touch refers to the client's willingness to be touched, the transparency of the motive behind the touch, and the requirement that the goal of the touch should be the client's well-being.
>
> **Non-maleficence** refers to the avoidance of causing harm by touching.
>
> **Beneficence** is a positive right of the client. It obliges professionals to always evaluate solutions from the point of view of the client's good, and to put the client's interests first in all situations. The principle of beneficence also requires the professional to be able to govern their own emotions and transfer positive and affirmative feelings to clients through touch.
>
> **Justice** means the equal right either to be touched or to refuse to be touched, according to the situation and the client's needs.

much pleasure as possible. A professional who takes a deontological approach touches their client because they consider touching to be inherently right or good in principle, irrespective of the consequences.

Kantian-oriented professionals decide how to touch another person by asking whether their manner of touching would constitute an acceptable universal principle for how people in general should touch each other. Immanuel Kant's categorical imperative demands that one should treat all people as ends in themselves, not as means to achieve one's own ends. There are actually three different formulations of the categorical imperative, the most famous being its formulation as a universal law:

Table 5.1 How theories of normative ethics align with professionals' questions about touch practices

Question about touching	Ethical theory
What is the purpose of touching? What are the consequences of touching?	Consequentialism
What kind of touch is right in itself? How would you like to be touched?	Deontology
How can touch benefit the maximum possible number of clients? How can touch be used as efficiently as possible?	Utilitarianism
Should I touch the client in the way I would want them to touch me? Is it possible to create general rules for professional touch that will be adequate in all situations?	Kantian ethics (categorical imperative)
What virtues are associated with touching? Is touching related to the character traits of the person who touches?	Virtue ethics
What kind of touch feels good to me?	Hedonism
Does the client have the right to be (or not to be) touched? Does everyone have an equal right to touch?	Rights

'Act in such a way that the maxim of any action could become a general law of nature by your will' (Kant, 2003). Virtue ethicists emphasise that virtues (e.g. kindness, discretion and vigilance) are associated with touching. They may also believe that a professional's habitual touch is closely related to their personal character traits or acquired skills. Virtue ethics thus emphasises moral characteristics, including practical wisdom (i.e. phronesis, discussed in Sect. 5.3). Virtue ethics was the dominant approach in Western moral philosophy up until the Enlightenment; it underwent an eclipse during the nineteenth century and then re-emerged in Anglo-American philosophy during the late 1950s (Hursthouse & Pettigrove, 2018).

Although the examples presented in Table 5.1 are somewhat banal, they illustrate the differences between normative ethical theories in relation to how touch as a moral action can be justified from various perspectives. Presumably, professionals sometimes justify their use of touch on the basis that it makes the client feel good (teleology). Sometimes, however, they may consider touch a duty because it represents what they regard as the right way of doing things (deontology). Professionals therefore rely on the moral principles described above, depending on the situation, even if they do not recognise the moral theories behind them.

5.3 Descriptive Ethics of Touch in an Organisational Context

Normative ethics and ethical guidelines strive to find proper justifications and guidelines for practical action, but in many respects, they remain abstract by comparison with the messiness of everyday working life. Non-normative ethics is therefore also needed in relation to touch—especially descriptive ethics, which can provide an understanding of the cultural and institutional settings in which touch occurs. While professionals need to know what kind of touch is justified and technically correct, promotes the client's good and well-being, or is in line with the goals of their work, mere technical skill or knowledge about ethical codes is not enough to ensure that physical contact is ethically sustainable. It is not enough for the touch to be performed in a correct and mechanically skilful way. The professional needs to recognise the multifaceted cultural meanings of gestures in order to be able to anticipate how the client will react. If the professional's motivation refers solely to the performance of an instrumental or protective touch, and not to a consideration of the client's needs, the professional may not only harm the client physically but also violate the boundaries of intimacy. Value awareness in touching includes a combination of technical, emotional and ethical skills that are materialised through the professional's presence and embodiment with the client.

The purpose of non-normative ethics is to describe what happens and how, and to examine the moral beliefs or arguments around the phenomenon in question. According to Beauchamp and Childress (2013), p. 2; see also Singer, 2011), descriptive ethics is a form of non-normative ethics because its objective is to establish what is factually and conceptually the case, not what ethically ought to be the case or what is ethically valuable. Descriptive ethics encompasses various orientations that take different perspectives on the cultural conditions, social values and organisational norms that guide how professionals touch clients. Professional ethics cannot only be about obeying the rules; it must also include critical thinking amid the crossfire of ethics, rules and conventions in relation to the rights and needs of clients, students or patients. Moral truths exist, but only real-life practice can reveal how they materialise in everyday activities. Touching is a living, intersubjective activity, so the development of different touch practices between people within an organisation makes the principles of ethical action visible, thereby also making them available for debate. We call this form of descriptive ethics 'embodied ethics': it is materialised through bodily interactions between people, so that values and attitudes—including appropriate and inappropriate ways to touch others –are negotiated as part of everyday situations.

Embodied ethics is a constantly changing set of practices that professionals adopt and modify with their clients and colleagues, partly consciously and partly unconsciously. Although Gerbert Sipman and colleagues (2019) do not use the term 'embodied ethics', their study shows how teachers use intuition in challenging situations where students have behavioural problems. The researchers call this skill 'pedagogical tact', which they define as 'teachers' ability to sense and act both swiftly and considerately in relation to large amounts of input at once' (Sipman et al., 2019, p. 1187). Intuition is not an unfounded belief about something but builds on prior knowledge and experience.

A more accurate term for intuition used by Sipman research partners (2019) is 'phronesis'. Phronesis is a kind of cultivated practical know-how. In *Nicomachean ethics*, Aristotle (1926) defines phronesis as 'a true and reasoned state of capacity to act with regard to the things that are good or bad for a man' (1104b5). As Rosalind Hursthouse and Glen Pettigrove (2018) put it, 'moral sensitivity, perception, imagination, and judgement informed by experience—phronesis in short—is needed to apply rules or principles correctly'. This means that knowing a set of rules or norms is insufficient. A person must also apply those rules in a way that is informed by the relevant features of the situation together with their experience. Only then will they have phronesis. A person who has phronesis can do two things. First, they can assess the situation in which they find themselves sufficiently accurately. This is the perception/sensitivity part. Second, they can use that assessment to decide what to do (Johnson, 2020, p. 228). In the case of touching, professionals might have embodied skills and know-how, but only after a degree of reflection and understanding regarding the situation can they engage with it in a proper manner. This practical know-how can be divided into three levels:

1. The professional has knowledge about the client's needs, social and health conditions, and rights, as well as an understanding of the organisation's values and touch culture.
2. The professional acquires the technical and ethical skills to touch in the right way and to constantly assess the consequences of their touch, and they are also ready to reflect on, change and adjust their touch according to the client's responses or behaviour.
3. The professional has the affective skill to convey the appropriate emotional state and atmosphere to the client through touch. If the professional lacks these affective skills, their touch may become mechanical and routine, and may not lead to the desired effects.

By adopting a reflexive attitude and listening to their clients, professionals can identify the ethical problems that arise in touch and devise appropriate solutions. For example, they will recognise that holding someone's hand can be variously interpreted as exerting power over the person, directing them, guiding them, forcing them in a particular direction, protecting them, encouraging them, paying attention to them, communicating with them, caring for them, worrying about them, stopping them, hurrying them along or even showing them love. Because of the ambiguity of touch, professionals usually verbalise their actions before they move; for example, before taking the client's hand, they may say, 'I'll hold your hand so that you don't fall' or 'I can't let you go there'. Speaking opens up the message conveyed by the touch, makes it visible and reinforces its reality. It helps others to perceive the embedded meaning of the touch. Treating the client's body with dignity, the professional also looks, touches and speaks in such a way that this dignity is realised in every situation. This sensitivity to the needs of others and the skill to express one's own perceptions, experiences, meanings and feelings as they arise through touch, is always in the best interests of the client.

Ethical principles related to touch practices are not implemented automatically, and a work community can activate values that distort the ethics of the activity. There may be hidden unethical practices that conflict with or even overrule the community's stated values. For example, a nursery school may state publicly that all parents should be equally involved in the development of the school's operations, and yet parents from cultural backgrounds that differ from those of employees may be overruled, or may not receive information about participation that is sufficiently clear or in their own language. Similarly, the relatives of residents in sheltered accommodation may be invited to participate in residents' care, but visiting restrictions imposed by the institution—for example, due to a pandemic—may prevent them from doing so, or professionals may communicate opposing opinions or values through their verbal expressions and bodily gestures. Indeed, hidden values are often stronger than official values. For example, there is research evidence that people with drug or alcohol abuse disorders, disabled people and older persons are discriminated against in treatment practices (Palukka et al., 2021). It is particularly detrimental to the realisation of clients' rights and dignity if an organisation's managers or supervisors do not intervene in—or even notice—the hidden values of their work community.

Of course, there are individuals who act unethically and unprofessionally towards their clients and colleagues, and this cannot simply be eradicated with good leadership. Unethical touch practices by a professional can include the intentional causing of pain, violent wrenching, neglect, sexual abuse, and at worst even killing. Often there are no witnesses to these kinds of touching. Thus, unethical touch between for example a teacher and a student, a police officer and a suspect, or a caregiver and a patient can be difficult to prove retrospectively. The burden of proof often falls on the victim. Breaches that involve touching a client in an unethical and damaging way are aggravated by the fact that the professional is always in a position of power in relation to the client. Thus, transparency in the transfer of knowledge in client work, and information about the organisation's values, can help professionals to act in accordance with their goals and responsibilities and to convey trustworthiness and competence to the client.

5.4   Facing the Other and Embodied Ethics

> I was treating a patient who had recently been moved to the hospice care unit for treatment because he could no longer cope with the palliative care he had been receiving at home, due to his increased restlessness and anxiety. One morning, when I went to his room, his anxiety was so strong that he was helpless; he stood by his bed on trembling legs and yelled incoherent words. I freaked out because I was afraid that he would fall and hurt himself. I rushed over to him, grabbed his shoulders with one hand to support him and took his hand in the other. We stood there, side by side, he a tall, wizened, trembling man, and me concentrating all my strength on not falling over. Based on the nonsense talk, I discovered he had existential and spiritual anxiety. I started talking to him calmly: 'I see that you are really anxious. Is there anything I can do to make you feel better?' While talking calmly, and assisted by another nurse, I directed him to sit on the edge of the bed and then on the far side. I stayed by his bed, talking quietly and stroking his hand while he relaxed and calmed down. He was not just a confused patient who needed sedative medication. He was a person at the end of his life, who longed to experience reconciliation and wholeness in his life. He also needed psychosocial conversational support. (Annu, one of us authors, who worked on a palliative care unit)

The passage quoted above—written by one of us authors—describes a situation where only a face-to-face encounter with a professional nurse can give comfort and confidence to a patient who is anxious about dying and pull them out of a panic attack. This example concretises how corporeal encounters are at the heart of the patient-professional relationship, although such encounters' unique meaning is often lost amid the demands of today's high-tech healthcare systems. To gain a deeper understanding of the meaning of corporeal encounters in healthcare, medical humanities scholars have explored Emmanuel Levinas' (1905–1995) writings on ethics (Edgoose & Edgoose, 2017; Tiemersma, 1987). According to Levinas, there is a unique responsibility and potential for hope that can only be found in corporeal—in this case, literally face-to-face—encounters.

Levinas' understanding of face-to-face interactions can be used to formulate a simple description of the everyday situation where a healthcare professional and a patient meet in the same room to address the patient's health concerns. Levinas argues that we should feel responsibility for even the smallest face-to-face interactions. A face-to-face encounter starts when we look at a person who looks back at us. In this kind of encounter, we face the other person by looking into their eyes, without seeing their face as an object. Levinas puts this as follows:

> You turn yourself toward the Other as toward an object when you see a nose, eyes, a forehead, chin, and you can describe them. The best way of encountering the Other is not even to notice the colour of his eyes! (Levinas, 1985, p. 85)

Levinas states here that we should refrain from looking at another person as an object. Consequently, he argues that the moment of facing the Other is always ethically compelling. Although the codes of professional ethics suggest rational rules regarding the extent of one's responsibility to patients to protect one from personal liability, Levinas reminds us that a face-to-face encounter is something far more complex and profound (Edgoose & Edgoose, 2017). Facing the patient awakens the professional's sense of responsibility and desire to help, but it also creates contradictions, and this is problematic for clinicians who want to keep their multiple patient relationships under control and who focus only on following rules and achieving results. Certainly, professionals are expected to use their expertise and knowledge to provide evidence-based interventions and rational advice to treat the patient. In the end, however, the outcome cannot be guaranteed, and professionals are fighting against the inevitable (such as illness or death) in their face-to-face interactions. Levinas argues that we do not *choose* to be responsible; indeed, in most cases we want to avoid responsibility if possible. But responsibility arises before we even begin to think about it, as if elicited by the approach of another person.

Although researchers into professional ethics have been inspired by Levinas' philosophy, his approach seems to be largely heuristic and too abstract to apply to the role of embodiment or touch in professional-client interactions (e.g. Nordtug, 2015). This is the conclusion reached by Michael Morgan (2007), who points out that Levinas works at a pre-theoretical and embodied level that represents the impetus behind ethical systems, which are forged through reflection, tradition and critique. If ethics refers to a study or system of moral principles, then Levinas approaches those principles only at a pre-theoretical and embodied level (Bergo, 2019). Rather than formulating an ethical theory, Levinas' discussion of the face-to-face encounter is relevant to contemporary ethics insofar as ethics is concerned with its own grounding in intercorporeality and sensibility. Nonetheless, there are parallels between Levinas and some contemporary ethical theorists. For example, moral intuitionists such as David Wiggins (1998) and John McDowell (1998) similarly focus on the role of sensibility in moral distinctions between right and wrong. Discussing education, McDowell (1998) argues that the acquisition of an ethical sensibility makes it possible for us to intuit what is right and good. However, there are very few ethical theories in which embodiment and intercorporeality are the focus.

Drawing on Merleau-Ponty's (1962/1989, 1968) philosophy, it is possible to formulate and examine guidelines for embodied ethics from the point of view of the virtues, duties or moral rules of professional touch. The ethical importance of Merleau-Ponty's work for professionals and work organisations rests, as Küpers (2015, p. 32) puts it, 'both upon the account he provides of the relational, bodily nature of the primordially inter-connected selves as mind-bodies and in their ambiguity, openness, creativity, and transcendence of relations involved.' Merleau-Ponty did not develop an embodied ethics as such, but the ethical importance of his work is based on the fact that he presents bodies as interconnected. Embodied ethical principles cannot be separated from cultural and institutional practices. With the help of Merleau-Ponty, we can interpret the body and embodiment as 'actors' or 'subjects' that are ethically reflexive and morally responsive in interactions between professionals and clients (see Box 4.1). Merleau-Ponty's phenomenological approach can help us to grasp the nexus of individual bodies and embodiment in relation to professional practices and touch cultures in work contexts. This also avoids the development of restrictive moral codes regarding how professionals are allowed to touch clients, or sets of business ethics that prioritise instrumentally oriented activities (Hancock, 2009; Ladkin, 2015). An embodied ethics approach can promote performative and ethically reflexive practice in and on action in relation to touch. This corporeal approach can help us to reconnect material properties (e.g. technologies) with experiences of ethical practice as part of our work organisation's culture (Styhre, 2004).

Embodied ethics can be considered a form of descriptive rather than normative ethics, since it does not provide strict answers about right and wrong. From a phenomenological perspective, embodied ethics can be seen as an emergent activity of bodily subjects and embodied intersubjective and corporeal processes in which professionals and clients are always already situated and actively participating in interaction (Küpers, 2012). Accordingly, embodied ethical subjects are culturally situated in continuous sensory ways—tactile, visual, olfactory or auditory. These incarnated subjects are exposed corporeally to whatever they perceive, feel, think, intend, do, make sense of or cope with morally, and they process it through their practices (Küpers, 2015). This embodied ethics requires genuine recognition of the Other—which includes other people, animals, artefacts and the environment—as both different and intrinsically valuable. What is ethically valued needs to be rooted in everyday life, and moral practices require us to empathise with and relate sustainably to other humans and non-human species.

As stated in Sect. 5.2, one of the core issues of professional ethics revolves around when and what kind of touch is morally right or wrong. Touch creates moral dilemmas and powerful, sometimes confusing feelings, but so does the avoidance of touch. Hence, abstaining from touch is not a solution to the moral dilemmas surrounding touching. During tactile contact, various emotional expectations arise that in themselves constitute an affective bond between people. People anticipate a possible touch, and they must deal with the feelings and sensations that arise during and after the touch. Through touch, an affective bond of some quality is formed between the professional doing the affective work and the client, and this bond can range from a cold and official relationship to a close and personal one. Touch sometimes 'glues' the professional and the client together, at least for the duration of the client relationship. Regardless of whether the professional or the client touches the other actively or passively, the touch always evokes affects in both parties. The power of touch in client work stems from this inevitable reciprocity of touch.

In his work *Visible and invisible*, Merleau-Ponty (1968) considers how touching and being touched are inevitably intertwined: one cannot touch something or somebody without simultaneously being touched. This 'double feeling' or reversibility between touching and being touched is one of the main themes in *Visible and invisible*, a collection of unfinished manuscripts and working notes published posthumously. Ultimately, we find a relationship of reversibility within the senses per se. In order to see, my body must be part of the visible and capable of being seen; likewise, in order to touch something or someone (or oneself), one's living body must be capable of being touched. In a famous example, Merleau-Ponty describes how when the right hand touches the left, the right hand is the toucher (active) while the left is the touched (passive) (e.g. Merleau-Ponty, 1968, pp. 139–149). In a way, one's own body is both the active toucher and the touched simultaneously. Nonetheless, the touching (right) hand can be reversed into a passive touched thing, while the (left) hand can be reversed into something active. Merleau-Ponty's concept of reversibility is important for thinking about professional touch. Whenever we touch someone, we are also touched by them; at the same time, the initially passive touch (i.e. being touched) can also become active.

However, reversibility does not entail a strict symmetry between touching and being touched. This is quite clear in everyday life: we do not assume that our touch intentions or touch acts evoke the same feelings in the other person as they do in us. Indeed, sometimes it is exactly the opposite: a touch given with good intentions can be experienced as oppressive by the recipient. Similarly, a light, distracted and unintentional touch can evoke deep emotions in the other person. Merleau-Ponty (1968) argues that the sentient and the sensible (i.e. touching and being touched) never wholly coincide but are always separated by a gap or divergence (*écart*) that defers their unity. For Merleau-Ponty, there is always already the mutual fluidity of reversibility and an ambiguous interplay between how one touches and how the other feels that touch, without collapsing into the similarity between touching and being touched. Even when I touch my left hand with my right, there is a gap between the two that makes my left hand an object for the right hand.

Formulating embodied ethics principally as an activity rather than a static system of moral codes allows us to consider responsiveness as a significant dimension of the ethics of professional touch. Phenomenologically, responsiveness comprises manifold interpretations of touching and receiving touch, including proactive orientation to another's touch, i.e., a readiness to being touched. Importantly, this response is processed by bodily senses, spatial orientations, gazes, gestures and desires, as well as memories and expectations with regard to professional tasks, work practices and organisational touch cultures. When responding to touch, we might be incited, attracted, threatened, challenged or appealed to by something or somebody. This affective state happens before we are able to take any deliberate initiative, aim at something or apply certain norms. This also makes the use of touch as part of professional work very challenging, even morally risky. Strictly speaking, it is difficult for professionals to 'use' touch, because they can never be completely sure how the client will respond to the touch. However, for practical purposes, we can talk about the 'usage' of touch, considering professional touch as a deliberative act and skilful action.

When professionals use touch in their work practices, their gestures always constitute both a response and a stimulus to clients. Touch invites, awakens, provokes or inspires the client—even when their response is not to touch. Canadian philosopher Erin Manning (2007) points out that precisely because of the reciprocity of touch, there is no such thing as touching—or in some cases not touching—without consequences. A touch seems to oblige us to react in some way. When a professional touches a client, the professional is themselves touched and moved by the tactile contact with the client, even if the client does not actively touch back. From the point of view of professionalism and professional coping, an important question is how the employee is able to regulate their own affects and the atmosphere of the tactile encounter. We will return to this question later, but first we will take a closer look at the three main values in touch practice: presence, sensitivity and empathy.

5.5 Presence, Sensitivity and Empathy

An early childhood educator summed up the most valuable task of her work as follows: 'Responding to the children's needs, it's truly our work' (Puroila et al., 2018). A practical nurse we interviewed who worked in elderly care described the essence of her work as 'comforting, presence and empathy—that is what we are also trained for'. A nurse in Benner's (2004) study also noted that being present was more effective than using physical restraints: 'Usually kind, gentle words, and caresses, and giving them the understanding that they're safe and healing seems to work'. These examples demonstrate that professionals perceive presence, sensitivity and empathy as core tasks of care work that are also efficacious in practice. Moments of encounter can provide a professional with an opportunity to notice the client's needs, give them hope, strengthen their dignity and help them to find their own resources.

Martin Buber's (1878–1965) philosophy of dialogue and presence can be used to concretise Levinas' philosophy (see Sect. 5.4): how can we face the Other without an objectifying gaze? Buber (1993) makes a distinction between the 'I-Thou' (*Ich-Du*) relationship and the 'I-It' (*Ich-Es*) relationship. I-Thou (or 'I-You') is a relationship that stresses the mutual, authentic existence of two beings, with neither being making any qualification or objectification of the other. There is no role in this relationship for imagination or opinion about the other being. But while the I-Thou relationship is an encounter between two beings, in the I-It relationship, by contrast, the beings encounter only mental representations (e.g. stereotypes) created and sustained by each individual mind. This means that the 'I' confronts and qualifies an idea or conceptualisation of the other being and treats that being as an object. If we apply Buber's concepts to the case of professional touch, an encounter on the I-Thou level requires the professional to give up their stereotypes and prejudices about the client, as already discussed in the context of multicultural encounters (see Sect. 3.5).

Typically, I-It situations are encounters where the professional touches the client in objectifying, routine, controlling, cynical or insensitive ways. Such encounters might include situations where a teacher angrily issues commands to their students in class, an early childhood educator ignores the rights of the family of a child from a different cultural background, a doctor does not discuss alternatives with the patient or a caregiver roughly pulls an elderly person out of a chair. In an I-It encounter, the professional's actions are not guided by the pursuit of the client's interests. Instead, for example, they might be guided by the professional's own emotions, their wish to perform a task assigned to them by a superior or related to their job description or obligations, or their desire to signal their own excellence or self-development. In addition, Buber (1993, p. 12) warns that if we always encounter other people in I-It relationships, we will gradually lose contact with our own self as well. Buber's strict division of interaction relationships into two types does not provide the professional with many opportunities to succeed, because creating a completely authentic relationship with a client depends on the skill and commitment of the professional's presence and awareness.

According to Buber, an I-Thou encounter entails *reaching out to someone for their sake*—which might also be a suitable slogan for good client work. Most often, professionals actually encounter their clients in I-It relationships, although even in these cases it is possible to build a respectful formal interaction with the client. However, it is not possible to achieve authenticity in such situations: the client is an externality, just one among many other clients, a number in a queue. The encounter does not take place in a manner that considers the client as an individual person.

The interaction between a professional and a client can also be understood as a form of co-presence: a living and non-discrete relationship between two individual subjects. Professionals do not see clients as rigid stereotypes, but treat them as people who are engaging in a dialogue that goes back and forth in an undefined way. Guindon et al. (2017) and Horton et al. (1995) state that touch is generally beneficial to the client when the client feels in control of the touch, and when the intervention meets the client's needs instead of the needs of the professional. In co-presence, both parties recognise and respect their roles and do not treat each other as objects.

5.5 Presence, Sensitivity and Empathy

The co-presence relationship between the professional and the client demands a lot of effort from the professional, whose work faces many time pressures. Nonetheless, the professional chooses their own way of encountering the client, regardless of whether it lasts for 20 seconds or 20 minutes, and whether it takes place as I-Thou or I-It. Being present means being available and taking a sensitive service attitude: I am here right now for you, and the duration of our encounter does not matter:

> The present is not fugitive and transient, but continually present and enduring. The object is not duration, but cessation, suspension, a breaking off and cutting clear and hardening, absence of relation and of present being. The beings are lived in the present, the life of objects is in the past. (Buber, 1993, p. 18)

Buber also underlines that it is only in the I-Thou relationship that the person is autonomous and thus able to choose how they encounter other people. In an I-It encounter, autonomy does not always materialise, and the professional may not have the opportunity to choose the circumstances—for example, if they are in a rush. In addition, professionals are using more and more technologies and devices, which sometimes make it difficult to create embodied contact with the client. In Sect. 4.3 we described digital distance as a zone where people who are physically close to each other do not communicate because they are on the internet, chatting on the phone or using some other technology or app. The central problem of digital distance is that the professional is not present to the client, even though they are physically sitting next to them.

So, what is presence, especially today, when it has become common to talk about telepresence in the context of remote and virtual technologies? Presence, being-with or being-available are indispensable aspects of human relations in general. From the perspective of embodied ethics, presence refers to an awareness of how one's own embodiment is situated and connected to other beings and the environment. Phenomenologically speaking, presence can include different conditions, starting from being merely physically present in a certain place at a certain time (as when students announce they are 'present' because they are not physically absent from class) to being mindfully present in one's own whole body (as in meditation practices). Often our presence falls somewhere between mere physical presence and full mindful presence, and it may also change from one moment to another. The term 'telepresence' was coined in 1980 by Marvin Minsky, who used it to refer to remote object manipulation applications and their teleoperation systems (Campanella, 2000). A branch of human-computer interaction research known as presence studies focuses on how an agent that is physically absent can have an impact on a certain location (see our discussion of telesurgery in Sect. 4.6), or how technology can create a simulation (i.e. virtual reality) of a setting that is not present. However, presence studies rarely discuss what presence really is or how technologies affect the experience or feeling of presence.

In the professional context, presence is by nature an intentional and concrete activity, and it involves skills that can be acquired. If they are attuned and present, professionals have the opportunity to identify the client's needs and find meaningful alternatives. They also have the opportunity to promote the good of the client. Touching in client work is not really possible unless one attunes oneself to the client's position and thus develops a co-presence with them. The ability to touch in an ethically approved manner is usually related to the individual's virtues and character strengths. A virtue, as Zagzebski (1996, p. 104) points out, is often perceived as a 'deep quality of a person, closely identified with her selfhood'. Once a virtue develops, 'it becomes entrenched in a person's character and becomes a kind of second nature' (Zagzebski, 1996, p. 116). Virtue can thus be considered a sensitivity or skill that can be cultivated. Being present and achieving co-presence with the client are virtues that can be cultivated.

Being present manifests itself in multiple ways, depending on the profession. For example, in the theatre, according to acting teacher Judith Weston (1996), presence makes the actor alert and sensitive both to their colleagues onstage and to the audience's receptivity and reactions to the actor's expressions. Although primary school teaching and theatre acting are very different professions, there are similarities in the meaning of presence in both cases. Like an actor, a teacher can best be present when they are relaxed, alert and confident. A professional in this state reacts sensitively to the students' expectations and feelings and is able to act confidently. A teacher who is tense, uncertain, stressed or immersed in their own thoughts does not evoke the experience among students that the teacher is there for them—even if the teacher is physically standing in front of them.

A professional is present when they speak in their own voice and inhabit their own skin instead of sticking rigorously to their formal professional role all the time. When a professional speaks in their own voice, the client who looks into their eyes can be sure there is somebody there. The professional's readiness for a dialogic encounter is transmitted to the client through their calm presence. The client feels safe if they sense that the professional is available and there for them. This is extremely important in end-of-life care, for example, both for the dying person and for others involved in the situation (see Haho, 2017; Haho, 2020). Quiet co-presence with the dying person is considered to be part of end-of-life care. Likewise, professionals who work with clients that have psychological problems need to have a special ability to be present. It is also difficult to imagine how professionals who work with children and young people might succeed in their tasks without genuine presence.

When the professional tunes into the other person's situation, tactile interaction becomes more than a mechanical routine. Through presence, it is possible to register the client's various emotions, feelings and bodily states, such as rejection, dissatisfaction, hostility, suffering, pain, depression or loneliness. Recognising these bodily reactions and states helps the professional to provide support for the client through the right kind of touch and other gestures. Thus, presence and sensitivity are value-based skills that are essential for identifying and responding to the client's needs. When the professional has the desire and opportunity to encounter the client at the I-Thou level, they can recognise nuances in the client's condition that cannot be measured or demonstrated with technological devices. By being present and

5.5 Presence, Sensitivity and Empathy

encountering the client, the professional is also able to sense the client's strengths and prioritise problems that do not need to be solved immediately.

Being present is closely connected to empathy, which refers to the ability to put oneself in another person's shoes. Empathy is often thought to be a character trait or emotion, but the German philosopher Edith Stein (1891–1942) suggested that empathy (*Einfühlung*) should be understood as an action or activity rather than an emotional state. In her doctoral thesis, published in 1917, Stein examined empathy as a skill that could be honed and developed. If we can put ourselves in another's shoes, we will see more clearly how their situation differs from our own habits and ways of looking at things. According to Stein (1989), empathy should not be equated with sympathy. Sympathy is often about top-down pity. In client work, professionals can put themselves in the client's position and assess how the client feels and how the professional should take those feelings into account. During an interview, one palliative care patient that empathy was exactly what she needed, and she felt this strongly in her body in treatment situations:

> It's not, it wouldn't feel very comfortable to me if I'm a case where the blanket is taken off in the morning and there's one person or another walking around in it, and that I am a case that it takes ten minutes to take care of and you have to get on your feet, I would then feel that I wouldn't want to be in that body at that moment, that I'm somewhere else, that I want to pretend I don't exist, so I wouldn't be here. (Reetta, Finnish 57-year-old female patient in hospice care unit)

However, it is clear that a professional can never fully reach the client's inner experience or claim to know how they feel. If a professional thinks they fully understand a client's feelings, they can all too easily start patronising the client. However, drawing on Stein's concept of empathy, Parviainen (2003) suggests that it is possible to formulate a special kind of empathy called 'kinesthetic empathy' (see also Brandstetter et al., 2013; Foster, 2010). Parviainen calls Stein's notion of empathy with another's experience 'empathising': when we put ourselves in another person's shoes, it can be as if we feel the other person's movements and gestures in our own body—we recognise the other's experience of sensations, movements and body positions. Seeing a woman who is pregnant, for example, women and men alike can empathise and thereby experience in their own bodies what it feels like to be pregnant, even if they have never experienced pregnancy themselves. Similarly, it is important for a physiotherapist or massage therapist to notice what positions or movements cause the client pain by empathising kinaesthetically with the client's lived body. One can hone one's ability to empathise kinaesthetically by doing various physical exercises, such as paying attention to the experiences evoked by positions, movements and movement qualities in one's own body.

A possible criticism that can be made of the embodied ethics of touch concerns the danger of idealism. Embodied ethics posits an ideal world where touch is beneficial through presence, and where the professional's organisation has no contradictions, conflicts or hierarchical power structures. In an ideal world, the importance of presence, sensitivity and empathy would be understood, absorbed and used with the greatest diligence by professionals, who would all use touch in beneficial ways for their clients. However, there are many grey areas and opportunities for abuse, and these deserve more attention within clinical practice, professional ethics and scientific research in the field of therapeutic touch.

Without the support of their organisations, managers and collegial communities, professionals may find it difficult to identify abuse situations and to follow the core values of the embodied ethics presented above. Organisations that recognise their employees as corporeally engaged beings within their occupational milieus also understand that embodied ethical dimensions play an important role in employees' work practices (Hockey & Allen-Collinson, 2009). Through embodied practice work and sense-making, embodied practitioners in organisations create, manage, reproduce, negotiate, interrupt and/or communicate somatic sensations and meanings that are related to client work and potential ethical concerns, including right and wrong touching (Küpers, 2015). This circumstantial and circumspection orientation is even more relevant in today's organisations, which are increasingly complex and heterogeneous, often producing paradoxical dilemmas in individual and collective settings. Next we turn to the limitations of using touch at work, especially with regard to clients who are unable to give their consent.

5.6 Dignity and Value Awareness with Vulnerable People

Ultimately, the need to be present is related to the need to meet the client respectfully and understand their dignity. The principle of respect for human dignity has strong historical and philosophical roots. Dignity seems to be part and parcel of fundamental human rights such as the right to life, equality, peace, health, self-determination and solidarity. Understanding dignity means recognising that people possess special value that is intrinsic to their humanity, and that they are worthy of respect simply because they are human beings. The ability to perceive and recognise others' dignity can be gained by unconscious learning, but a professional can also actively cultivate this ability—for example, through presence.

The cherishing of dignity provides a value-based foundation for professional touch that combines honour, safety, trust, willingness to negotiate, community, loyalty, solidarity, care and responsibility (e.g. Rónay, 2019). From this perspective, professional practice is not to be understood as an isolated performance or the fulfilment of a duty, but as a comprehensive attitude to life: a desire to encounter others and promote good by respecting human dignity. Because dignity can all too easily remain an abstract concept, we provide some examples from our own interview material of how nurses who worked in end-of-life care described respect for dignity as an embodied quality (see also Kinnunen et al., 2019). In end-of-life care, the professional's ability to touch the patient can provide comfort and create supportive conditions for a peaceful ending. In Box 5.2, we present five core principles of touch that our interviewees proposed to convey respect for the dying person's dignity, along with interview extracts that illustrate how those principles can be embodied through touch.

> **Box 5.2 Dignity Materialised as Presence and Touching Between Practical Nurses and Elderly People in End-of-Life Care**
>
> **Sit near an unconscious patient:** Then it changes in such a way that the presence, and the fact that we constantly try to communicate by touching, or a nurse can sing or speak, that there is someone present, no one has to die alone. Even though it feels as if I can't see anything from there, this person is dying and going now, despite that, they need the person present. (Hilkka, Finnish practical nurse)
>
> **Focus on one's co-presence with the patient:** It becomes even more considerate, calmer, gentler, when we try to make those last moments as good as possible and as painless, gentle, peaceful as possible. Yes, it changes the tone of the touch completely. And it changes for everyone, even though nothing is ever said about it, so when the doctor says or makes a note that there is hospice care, we start the hospice care, then everyone's style changes. I'm not the same kind of nurse, I've worked with a change in style. Somehow that kind of appreciation of life comes out more clearly. (Sirkka, Finnish nurse)
>
> **Do not rush when co-caring for a patient:** The situation is always trying to calm down, so that there is no rush to take any measures. When washing them or dressing them or doing some procedure or performing oral care for them, just such basic things. So, it's done in such a way that there's usually a lot of teamwork involved, so that there's not much one person can do, like washing their face, wiping their mouth, things like that. You don't have to pull or push anything, and that way the movements are calm. (Vilma, Finnish practical nurse)
>
> **Do not leave patients alone:** Yes, more comprehensive than that, yes. Of course, there are words, and we are guided verbally, it's not 'what we are going to do now?' Posture therapy, however, in a central sense, and in pain management, if only that's it. And then really that touch is more too, it can be for example that their feet are massaged, and their hands are massaged, depending on which stage of hospice care we are going to, but that it is a more holistic touch. We have agreed that we will not be alone, so that it will be as good as possible for the resident. So that he doesn't have to support anything himself at any point, that it will be as painless and pleasant as possible. (Rebekka, Finnish practical nurse)
>
> **Do not use gloves:** Probably, probably it will be emphasised even more that it is taken more gently. And of course, without those gloves, if it's at all possible that you can handle the dying resident. Yes, there will be, quite clearly you will be even more careful when it is a fragile person, however, all those turning situations and all that, you don't think about how you will catch that person. Yes, it [the touch] is highlighted. (Liisa, Finnish practical nurse)

Value awareness means the professional's ability to understand the professionally validated knowledge, principles, values and beliefs that govern their practice, especially when they are encountering a client in a vulnerable situation (e.g. Milliken, 2018; Holopainen et al., 2014; Sayers & de Vries, 2008). Baruch Fischhoff and Amber E. Barnato (2019, p. 5), who have studied value awareness in decision-making in end-of-life care, define the concept as 'recognizing, addressing, and, perhaps, accepting situations where people do not know what to think or want'. They suggest that with a vulnerable client, a competent professional may find it difficult to find a balance between scientific knowledge, collegial suggestions, standard ethical options and their own emotions. However, they can develop value awareness to find that balance when offering support to the client, 'to achieve their desired balance between rational and non-rational decision making, allowing them to be as rational as they can and want to be' (Fischhoff & Barnato, 2019, p. 2). Fischhoff and Barnato urge professionals to rely on their own value awareness rather than on rationality in end-of-life care situations. Value awareness in end-of-life care is related to the patient's experience of a holistic encounter; caring; autonomy; relief for their symptoms, distress and loneliness; respect; being human, and being themselves; meaningful relationships; and dignified treatment (e.g. Bylund-Grenklo et al., 2019; Fischhoff & Barnato, 2019; Guo & Jacelon, 2014; Hemati et al., 2016). The value awareness of the patient's family members reveals itself in practices that enable the dying person to live as a respected human being in relation to self and others, to maintain their identity, to feel connected to their significant others, and to be comfortable with their new situation (Sandgren et al., 2020).

Many healthcare professionals also face situations where it is necessary to avoid touching a vulnerable client. Norris et al. (2003) indicate that therapists should avoid touching clients who have undergone a recent trauma where their boundaries were transgressed or even violated. Such clients also tend to be severely self-critical and prone to feelings of shame. They experience intense emotions in the therapeutic relationship, and they may confuse the closeness of the relationship with love. Moreover, therapeutic touch does not produce favourable results with clients who tend to hand over total power to the psychotherapist, or conversely with clients who try to dominate the relationship. Warnecke (2011) points out that psychotherapists' supervisors must pay special attention to the risk of collusion with the client when therapeutic touch is used, which often leads to a loss of objectivity towards the client. The risk is that the touch will create a strong bond, perhaps leading the therapist to reinforce emotions that are harmful to the client.

Moral sensitivity in professional decision-making and actions comes especially to the fore in situations where the client lacks full capacity—for example, if they are very young, have a memory impairment or mental illness or are unconscious. In addition to these cases, researchers Bettina Stenbock-Hult and Anneli Sarvimäki (2011) highlight the issue of shared vulnerability. This issue concerns both parties in the encounter and is a resource as well as a burden: vulnerability is based on openness and authenticity, but it may also entail weakened capacity or resilience, suffering in the wake of life events, or poor skills to cope with everyday tasks. Many researchers (Altintas et al., 2022; Bergen, 2020; Mo & Shi, 2021; Shaukat et al.,

2020) have reported increased vulnerability especially in elderly care. Both residents and staff in nursing homes suffer from emotional exhaustion, loneliness, uncertainty, hopelessness, work overload and role conflicts. However, trust diminishes the fear of vulnerability. Trust evokes a sense of security in people, and they can be more relaxed in the face of an encounter.

5.7 Ethics of Non-touch Policies

As previously stated, psychoanalysts and psychotherapists (other than body therapists) may feel reluctant to touch their clients in any manner, although connecting touch is used by psychiatric nurses in particular to build supportive and trusting relationships with patients (see Sect. 2.1.1). In psychoanalysis, for example, it is assumed that therapeutic touch would contaminate the transference relationship between analyst and patient, disturbing the analysis and even running the risk that the therapist's personal satisfaction will be prioritised over the client's psychological well-being (Johnston & Farber, 1996). For these reasons, many people might be surprised to hear that Sigmund Freud touched his patients when he met them in his consulting room, sometimes massaging or touching their heads (Guindon et al., 2017). Because Freud wanted psychoanalysis to be perceived as an objective science, he gave up the practice of therapeutic touch (Phelan, 2009). Ever since then, both psychoanalysts and psychotherapists have been wary of all uses of touch in their practice.

Nowadays, the fear of being accused of sexual misconduct is the principal reason why many psychotherapists prefer to abstain from any form of touch (Norris et al., 2003; Phelan, 2009). According to Harrison and colleagues (2012), mental health professionals have stopped all discussion surrounding the theme of therapeutic touch for fear of being accused of sexual misconduct by their clients. Although the benefits of touch have been the topic of many studies, and there is evidence of the therapeutic value of touch in psychotherapy (Bonitz, 2008; Harrison et al., 2012; Phelan, 2009; Westland, 2011; Zur, 2007), many psychotherapists perceive it as too risky. These psychotherapists believe that touching the client cannot be an ethically sustainable practice because there have been some cases of sexual misconduct in psychotherapy. However, touch can have a reassuring effect on the psychotherapeutic client, increasing their engagement in the therapy, leading them to perceive the psychotherapist as trustworthy, and making it easier for them to open up (Guindon et al., 2017). Mic Hunter and Jim Struve's (1998) study found that touch could establish, maintain and even deepen the therapeutic alliance between client and psychotherapist.

Similarly, as discussed in Sect. 3.4, early childhood education professionals and primary school teachers consider that touching a child may be perceived as sexual in tone, especially when the professional in question is male (see also Alexander, 2001; Stover & Carlson, 2006). Teachers are unsure whether their touch might be taken to signal something unethical, and this leads them to reflect deeply on their own intentions and motives, or even to consciously avoid touching children. This generalised 'no-touch' policy may be reinforced by the implicit practices of co-workers: for example, when a female teacher looks worriedly at a male colleague who is about to hug a crying child, she sends him an implicit message about untouchability (Stover & Carlson, 2006). No-touch policies formulated by schools or other authorities can take the form of restrictions—for example, teachers might be advised to hug a child from the side instead of from the front, or to offer them a high five instead of a hug. Judith Duncan's (1999) study reveals the effects of no-touch and sexual abuse protection policies on female teachers' work in early childhood education. As surveillance has increased, tensions have intensified between the teacher's own self-trust and the parents' perceived lack of trust. Duncan points out that anxiety about child abuse in educational institutions is not limited to male teachers and affects more and more female teachers too. Thus, holding a child in one's arms, which has been considered a fundamental factor in children's positive development, provokes fear and confusion among educators and teachers.

As Suzanne Imes (1998) reminds us, if early childhood education professionals or psychotherapists confine themselves to talking, and if they refuse to touch children, they may miss opportunities to allow clients to express certain emotions through touch—which is sometimes the only outlet available to them. In early childhood education, being hugged and held can be seen as the child's basic right and a prerequisite for their balanced mental growth and emotional life. Against this background, educators must weigh up the child's best interests and the available solutions for their well-being—that is, how to strengthen the child's dignity, humanity and right to well-being through touch. One might argue that early childhood education inevitably includes physical closeness along with other sensory contacts between the child and the educator.

In addition to professionals' various fears and the justified restrictions on touch in client-professional interactions, one's working conditions and available resources also limit the use of touch at work in multiple ways. The work of professionals is increasingly driven by the need to perform tasks more quickly or cost-effectively, or by the goal of achieving something other than a profound encounter with the client. This may lead to the reduction or elimination of touch, or to its use in hasty, harmful or even dangerous ways. In such extreme cases, the professional's action is guided by something other than a touch-promoting ethics or a respect for dignity. Several researchers (e.g. Kröger et al., 2019; Papastavrou & Suhonen, 2021; Sihto & Aerschot, 2021; Suhonen & Vaarto-Rajalin, 2021; Tistad et al., 2012) have stressed that cuts to public service funding, as well as care poverty because of a shortage of personnel or resources, are worrying current trends that threaten decent care practices. 'Care poverty' refers to the situation where older adults in particular receive inadequate care services to support their everyday activities, which at worst leads to violations of their basic rights. It can also refer to fully automated and mechanised care from which a nurse's touch and embodied presence have been eliminated.

We have seen how the COVID-19 pandemic resulted in the collapse of physical contact and touch between people. People had to avoid touching each other because of the risk of transmitting the virus. As well as isolating us from each other, COVID-19 also affected our experiences of safety and mental well-being.

Professionals experienced touch at work as a risk to their own or their family members' physical health, and this caused them high levels of depression, anxiety, insomnia and distress (e.g. Altintas et al., 2022; Bergen, 2020; Elbqry et al., 2021; Fernandez et al., 2020; Mo & Shi, 2021; Pype et al., 2021; Shaukat et al., 2020). The contradiction between professionals' perception of patients' needs for touch on one hand, and the practical restrictions that meant they could provide only gloved or technology-mediated instrumental touch on the other, led to ethical distress for many professionals. The prolonged precautionary measures made people realise the extent to which they had previously understood touch as a natural gesture of kindness and a prerequisite for trust. The prohibition on touch was a prohibition against demonstrating warmth towards the client and respect for their importance and dignity.

5.8 Rewarding Touch Intertwined with Professional Identity

The mastery of touch as a work skill is associated with the feeling of success at work. The ability to touch a client in reasonable and pleasant ways can take different forms in different professions, but many of the healthcare professionals we interviewed emphasised that they found it rewarding. Similarly, early childhood education professionals can feel deep satisfaction when they hold a child in their arms while dressing them and sensing that the child is thus receiving the caring adult touch they desperately need (Keränen, 2022). A teacher can relieve a student's restlessness and generally communicate human solidarity and care in the classroom through touch. Reciprocity and the experience of success alleviate the ethical distress that can arise at work.

Such rewarding experiences of the skilful use of touch during work routines are connected to and develop one's professional identity. Sometimes, creating a trusting working relationship with the client through touch takes time and stretches one's professional capacities to the maximum. When the connection is finally established in such cases, it is probably even more rewarding, and even more of a professional learning experience, than ordinary encounters. Conversely, a failure to create a trusting tactile connection can weaken the professional's sense that their work is meaningful and damage their confidence in their own abilities to work in challenging situations.

According to Naike Bochatay (2018, p. 263), professional identity is 'an individual's efforts to make their work meaningful to themselves, including the professional values that differentiate them from other groups'. When creating and reflecting on their professional identity, professionals ask themselves questions such as:

- Who am I?
- What do I understand, and how do I act?
- What are my tasks and duties?
- What information do I require in order to identify the client's needs and work accordingly?
- What are my decisions based on, and where would different choices lead?

One's professional identity is created in interaction with one's work community. This happens partly unconsciously as one adopts certain manners of working, including touch practices. At the same time, knowledge and practices shared by the working community are filtered through the professional's own morals and their conceptions of ideal practice. Thus, it can be said that professional identity consists in the professional's personal skill and their way of filtering their profession's goals and values into their own way of working; at the same time, it also represents the way the entire profession works and expresses its basic task priorities (Fitzgerald, 2020). During our interviews, practical nurses often reported that they had certain responsibilities that were related to their profession. Their identities included notions about good and correct ways of working linked to their profession, but also their own ethical solutions:

> So, it is part of the role of a practical nurse, which we have also been trained to do, which we also have to consider that it is not just a routine job of changing incontinence pads and giving food. It also involves psychological and social care, in my opinion. We come in many different types, but this is still such an important thing to me, because it makes me feel good if I have even been thanked by an older person for my care, or if that thanks comes in some other way. With a smile or similar, you know you've done a good job. From person to person. (Hilkka, Finnish practical nurse)

Studies in the field of education have found that a teacher's strong identity is connected to a commitment to their work and a confidence in their own abilities to do the work, develop and succeed in their career. An OECD Education Working Paper (Suarez & McGrath, 2022) examines the development of teachers' professional identities in different teaching environments and contexts. The information contained in the report is intended to be used not only within the profession or to develop education and research, but also for political decision-making. The report argues that demands and expectations are made of teachers' work in changing social environments:

> The roles of stakeholders have changed and diversified over time: parents, students, policy makers and other key actors from the community in general, such as the labour market and the research community, differ in the expectations they have towards schools. (Suarez & McGrath, 2022, p. 7)

It is interesting to note that the report understands teachers' professional identity as a flexible, dynamic and constantly evolving construct that demands reactions to the diverse, even contractionary expectations of different stakeholders. According to Valentina Suarez and Jason McGraths' (2022) summary of the report, teachers' professional identity is formed through the interaction between (1) the educational system and school context, (2) the structures and support of the education institution, (3) teachers' behaviours and attitudes, and (4) student outcomes. It is clear that any professional identity will be reconstructed by repeated responses to constantly changing circumstances and expectations, but perhaps this has applied particularly strongly to teachers in recent years.

To sum up, professional identity is a way of being and acting during work tasks, and it is formed through multifaceted individual and social factors and learning processes. Further, it is shaped by one's professional experience and career development. Through external signs—such as work clothes, or the 'choreography' of certain routine work practices—the professional expresses their status and the nature of their tasks. Through embodied gestures—nuances, rhythms and orientations—the professional holistically expresses their value commitments and fundamental conceptions: what I want to be, what I really am, and what I strive for. Besides the use of one's voice, facial expressions and movements, touch is a very concrete way to reflect one's embodied professional identity. Due to the reciprocity and affective nature of touch, the client is an intimate part of the experience and growth of the professional's identity; it is almost as if the client can feel it 'in their own skin'. To give an example, Anna-Maija Puroila and colleagues' insights into 'armchair pedagogy' perfectly describe this experience in early education. Educators and researchers in a Finnish preschool came up with an excellent pedagogical idea based on reciprocity and touch, which the educator Raisa explained as follows:

> This requires understanding that we must sit on the floor. Then we've the armchair, which is our best friend nowadays. We've permission to sit on the armchair and listen to the children. (Raisa, Finnish early childhood educator, quoted in Puroila et al., 2018, 25)

Armchair pedagogy as a method offers a safe and calm 'circumference' for the early childhood educator and the child. It consists of the present moment, close togetherness, and touching with the whole body. In terms of professional identity development, it underlines the educator's basic task and the values attached to it, and it offers a concrete way to embody it with children through touch and one's whole embodied being. In our own interviews, Sofia, who worked as a practical nurse in a long-term care unit, described how the development of her professional identity was closely linked to how she had learned to touch clients in the right way. The variety and range of her touches increased as her skills developed. In addition, she told us that work experience and age had given her the courage to use touch to comfort elderly clients or their relatives:

> I'm no longer as shy to touch as I was when I was younger. And of course, it probably depends on the situation, these are the old people who live here. When I was younger, when I worked in a different place, people were treated differently. But yes, I do notice that when I was younger, I probably wouldn't have hugged the relatives when their loved one died. Now it doesn't cause me any problems if they come to hug me, or I hug them. Of course, you always must think a little about whether – they like it, but if you've known someone for years, they usually like it that way. (Sofia, Finnish practical nurse)

In studies examining touch between elderly clients and their caregivers, it has been found that when they touch their clients consciously and thoughtfully, caregivers perceive themselves as valuable and competent professionals. Novice nurses feel empowered when they learn to ease their patients' suffering through touch. By successfully touching the client with a professional grip, the novice nurse feels physically that they are taking on the professional status of a nurse. As well as clients themselves, awareness of the presence and professionality of touch can also be very important for their relatives and friends, who will be concerned about the risk that their loved one might receive poor or inhumane care. Thanks received from the patient's nearest and dearest are thus rewarding for the professional. The rewarding feeling generated by reciprocity with clients and their loved ones is sometimes perceived as the main motivation for a nurse's work. One of our interviewees, who worked at a nursing home, stated that she was not motivated by monetary reward, even though 'it is necessary for my livelihood'; rather, the most important motivator for her was the gratitude she received from her elderly clients, their relatives and her own work community. By gratitude she meant not only spoken words but also situations—for example, when a client softly patted her hand as a sign of thanks for her gentle assistance with eating.

We conclude that skilful touch and sensitivity to the client's needs can increase the professional's psychical and physical resources at work and develop their professional identity. Being touched gives positive power to the client, which is then returned to the professional. The reciprocity of touch creates co-presence and cohesion, enabling mutual understanding even when there is no shared verbal language. This feeling is especially familiar to those who work in hospice or dementia care and who communicate a lot with their clients through touch. Rebekka who worked in geriatric ward summed this up:

> Professionalism is thought to mean that no emotional ties should arise, but perhaps a certain kind of togetherness. Especially if those words are not there, then the understanding that when I act like this, the other person reacts in this way. And this kind of togetherness encourages you to continue on the path of touching them. In my own work at the moment, it's precisely that calming down, usually getting a certain kind of contact, even some kind of touch. If you can't make eye contact any more, then touch them. However, that sense of connection remains until the end. (Rebekka, Finnish practical nurse)

Nevertheless, professionals often find themselves in conflicting situations where commonly agreed practices require rapid reconsideration and improvisation to act in appropriate ways. They may feel confused and uncertain, even doubtful or anxious about what to do. Professionals may then find themselves in confrontational situations where encountering or touching a client causes moral distress.

5.9 Moral Distress

Moral distress among professionals usually occurs in situations where they do not know the right way to touch or feel unable to resolve the dilemma based on their own moral choices. Andrew Jameton (1984) simply defines the emergence of a moral burden as a situation where a person experiences both a difficult moral situation and psychological stress and there is a causal connection between the two. Debra R. Hanna (2004), on the other hand, describes moral distress as an umbrella category that can include experiences of anguish or suffering associated with a moral dilemma, moral uncertainty or certainty accompanied by constraint. An ethical dilemma that requires a solution, as well as expectations regarding decision-making and choice, can lead to a moral distress when (1) the professional does not know the right way to act or (2) they do not act according to what they know to be the right way to act. Not choosing or ignoring the dilemma is also a choice or solution. The background may be the professional's inability to recognise ethical principles, which in turn causes confusion and can also lead to incorrect solutions. When a professional perceives a solution to be wrong or inappropriate, this also causes moral distress. Distress can also arise when the professional feels that for some reason they are being forced to act against their own values or notions of right and wrong.

In some situations, ethical decision-making can produce a cumulative problem known as 'moral hazard'. This describes a power differential between those who make decisions and those who must live with those decisions. Resource shortages in many service sectors have led to this difficult kind of moral problem. Studies have also shown that a higher level of moral distress often correlates with a poorer perceived ethical climate (Hamrick & Blackhall, 2007; Hamrick, 2014; Hanna, 2004). It also appears to be correlated with other experiences that have similar affects, such as compassion fatigue and burnout (Maiden et al., 2011; Rushton et al., 2015). These generate many follow-up ethical questions for professionals, to which there are not always clear and solid ethical answers. Solutions to emerging dilemmas are often sought collegially, which means that many relevant factors affecting the situation have to be weighed together.

Divergent conceptions of what constitutes appropriate touch, or what human dignity in all its nuances means, may cause tension or even conflict between a professional and their client. In addition, the client may sometimes lose control of their emotions and behave in a way that violates the rights or dignity of the professional or other clients. The professional's ability to react to the client's intentionally or unintentionally aggressive, sexually offensive or otherwise inappropriate touch is related in many ways to the professional's behaviour, various situational factors and how the organisation has prepared for such situations by providing resources, education and instruction. The professional has various resources to respond to the client's unethical touch without resorting to violent touch or retaliation.

Instead of setting out instructions or guidelines for how to act in unexpected situations, we will now reflect on clients' potentially dangerous behaviour with the help of two examples (Boxes 5.3 and 5.4). One resource available to professionals was introduced in Sect. 2.1.7; the professional can resort to a protective touch by pinning the client's arms, for example, and trying to keep them still, thereby protecting themselves and others from being hurt. With the two examples presented in Boxes 5.3 and 5.4, we draw on descriptive ethics to consider the kinds of ethical questions that can arise from the perspective of dignity and human rights in messy situations where one is using protective, controlling or distancing touch.

A professional should weigh up the extent to which it is justified to limit the rights of a boisterous child—for example, by restricting how they can move and play—in order to keep other children out of danger. A boisterous child who is not

> **Box 5.3 A Boisterous Child in a Day Care Group**
> A day care group comprises ten children aged between one and three years, one of whom is very boisterous. When the group is moving from one place to another—for example, when they are going for a walk or going out to eat—the general atmosphere among the children can be restless and fast-paced. The smallest children, who have only recent learned to walk, cannot move quickly, and they tend to fall over when the boisterous child gets excited. It seems that his emotional capacity is still undeveloped, and he lacks the skills to control his emotions, which produces dangerous situations for other children. The other children's parents are also worried about the behaviour of this boisterous child and the safety of their own children.
>
> Early childhood educators often have to forcibly take the boisterous child in their arms, thereby protecting the others until the transition has been peacefully completed. They also consider whether to isolate him in another room, away from the other children, during such transitions.
>
> From the point of view of professional ethics, we can discuss whether this procedure would constitute equal treatment of all the children. We can ask:
>
> 1. Is it right to give the boisterous child more space and the full attention of one educator when the other children have less space and only one educator between them?
> 2. Is it right to isolate the boisterous child from the other children if he does not understand the reason why he is not allowed to be with the others?
> 3. What are the ethical ways to calm the child down and guide him to become aware of his feelings and control his behaviour?

able to self-regulate their activity may experience such prohibitions and orders as unfair punishment. On the other hand, other children may become stressed by the activities of both a boisterous child and the educator who is in charge of that child. A professional needs to be able to manage the group dynamics so that no one suffers from the situation unreasonably. However, the available resources (staff numbers and facilities) in day care centres often limit the available solutions, and in many cases, all the parties involved end up suffering to a greater or lesser degree. This may lead to ethical distress for the professionals.

Sometimes, people with Alzheimer's disease or other memory impairments become upset or angry for no obvious reason. They may throw things, or resist their caregivers by pushing and hitting them. The reasons behind this 'aggressive' behaviour are unclear, but we can presume that the behaviour is not deliberate. Often the attacks flare up without warning, but there may be triggers that other people can spot before or during the outburst—for example, if the person is touched in an uncomfortable way, if they feel that their personal space has been invaded, or if there are loud noises or too much activity in their environment. In many cases, the resources (staff numbers, facilities) available in nursing homes are limited, which means that the nurses do not have sufficient oversight of the circumstances to

> **Box 5.4 A Violent Dementia Patient in Long-Term Residential Care**
> Old adults with various physical and mental impairments, including some people with memory disorders, live in a sheltered accommodation unit. One resident with dementia, a heavy woman in good physical condition, occasionally behaves violently towards others. Her behaviour is unpredictable: she is sometimes very kind, funny and considerate to her fellow residents and care providers, but she might suddenly hit the person in front of her for no apparent reason. The care staff must often intervene physically and control her to protect other residents and professionals. She clearly cannot control her impulses; her intention is not to cause harm on purpose. Presumably, she becomes anxious because there is someone in front of her against whom she feels she has to defend herself. Some of the other residents know how to watch out for her, but those with memory impairments in particular are not able to do so. Attempts have been made to adjust her medication, but the violent outbursts have not stopped.
>
> In consultation with one of her relatives, the care staff decide to limit this woman's freedom of movement in communal areas by locking her alone in her room on some occasions.
>
> We can consider whether this controlling practice follows sustainable professional ethics by asking the following questions:
>
> 1. What are the rights of the adult with dementia who has behaved violently?
> 2. Is limiting her freedom of movement right and respectful of human dignity, considering that other residents may be subjected to violence?
> 3. What are the ethical ways to calm a dementia patient down and control her behaviour?

protect the potentially violent client, or other residents or personnel, from these violent eruptions.

The work community should provide a safe space for professionals to talk openly about the moral distress they feel in different tactile encounters with clients. It is important for an individual employee to receive understanding and support from their colleagues and supervisors. Sometimes it is also constructive to reflect critically on one's own actions and reactions in an honest but supportive atmosphere. The goal should not be to evaluate the individual employee, but to support them to develop their professional attitude and manner of acting. Work communities benefit when each individual member is aware of the organisation's explicitly presented values and can safely reflect on their own ways of working in relation to them, even when it feels difficult. It should also be possible for individual employees to criticise the organisation's culture and to participate in its development. Moreover, it is important to be able to find solutions together for client encounters that are perceived as challenging. This can significantly facilitate the processing and management of emotions that arise in client encounters, and thus can benefit clients too.

Unfortunately, professionals can face inappropriate touching by clients. Studies have shown that nursing staff are in an especially vulnerable position regarding sexual harassment, and more research is needed on the topic (e.g. Grigorovich & Kontos, 2019; Nielsen et al., 2017). Sexual harassment involves the use of explicit or implicit sexual overtones in speech, touch and other gestures, and it occurs in various client work communities. The term 'sexual harassment' first appeared at the beginning of the 1970s, and it was especially highlighted by feminist activist Catharine MacKinnon at the turn of the 1980s. Although sexual harassment is illegal in many countries, sexual harassment laws generally do not prohibit minor isolated incidents. In the workplace, harassment may be considered illegal if it is frequent or severe and thereby creates a hostile or offensive work environment. Even though sexual harassment is quite common—for instance, in Germany and England, one in two women has experienced some form of sexual harassment, according to a Eurotrack survey (YouGov, 2020)—it is difficult for the victim to produce evidence that it has occurred. We have already noted that the power of the #Metoo campaign is making the problem ever more visible, and presumably also decreasing it.

Female nurses are more likely to become targets of sexual harassment than male nurses (Kahsay et al., 2020). In a harassment situation, a female nurse is treated as an object that can be sexualised and touched without permission. One interviewee who worked in home care told us about a case where a male client with dementia had repeatedly harassed all the female home care workers he encountered. According to her, the man clearly had a degrading attitude towards women: after getting to know his personal history, the staff drew the conclusion that all women were objects of contempt and subjugation for him, including his late wife. The man made sexual suggestions and insulted the women, and no one dared to let him stand behind them for fear of a sudden attack. The situation became burdensome for the workers, and attempts were made to ease it, for example by rearranging shifts. Male nurses, on the other hand, face a different burden produced by the sexualisation and gendering of touch: the burden of emotional work. Studies have shown that the touch of male nurses, teachers and athletics coaches in particular is dogged by the suspicion that their intentions are sexual, and this can be very frustrating and stressful for male workers (see Sect. 3.4).

As the #Metoo campaign and the COVID-19 pandemic have revealed, many global and societal norms and ways of behaving can change quickly when necessary. We have underlined how #Metoo and COVID-19 have deeply influenced how we think about touch. For instance, we may have become more careful about touching other people, started to avoid touch or changed some of our other touch habits. Despite their negative impacts on touch cultures, these worldwide phenomena have also had some positive outcomes: many people are much more aware of their way of touching than they were a few years ago. A touch that was previously perceived as routine suddenly demands attention. The global pandemic brought into focus the meanings and importance of touch in everyday interactions, and how crucial tactile contact is for multiple groups of clients. Many professionals have discovered how difficult their working conditions become if they have to consciously avoid touching clients or even objects. With the avoidance of touch, a part of the bodily message that conveys care, warmth, respect and care is lost.

Touch in client work is not only rewarding and empowering but can cause mental strain and moral distress. A professional's experiences and feelings related to touch can be unpleasant, disturbing or violating for many reasons. Professionals may find some clients more difficult or intimidating to touch than others. Sometimes touching the client's body feels unpleasant because of secretions, dirt, traces left by drug use, odour or other factors. In such cases it can be difficult for the professional to have a completely neutral attitude to touch, even if the client themselves arouses empathy and the desire to help (see Sect. 2.5). That is why professionals often hide such feelings not only from their clients but also from their colleagues. Furthermore, one's own touch can cause a reaction in the client, which is not desirable from the professional's point of view. As stated previously, our touch may not necessarily evoke the feelings in the other person that we intend. A client may perceive any kind of touch as threatening, which will make it much more difficult to perform a mandatory procedure, for example. The client may also be so reserved that professionals do not succeed in creating a connection with them through touch, despite their best efforts. This is especially problematic in client encounters where touch is the primary medium of communication, such as with small children and deafblind clients.

Professional activity is not an isolated performance or the fulfilment of a duty. It is a comprehensive attitude to life, a way of encountering others and promoting good by respecting human dignity. Although the core task of a professional is to promote dignity in every situation and in as many ways as possible, there is no list of right or wrong practices. Professionals seek to create dignity-based solutions in every single situation. Thus, they should always be interested in developing their own professional capacity and communication skills, and they should always be ready to accumulate evidence-based knowledge, understand their own interpretations and experiences and reflect on ways to convey sensitivity in general. Both sides in a tactile contact interpret the encounter from their own horizons, based on their unique life courses and circumstances. Nonetheless, it is important to develop a shared understanding of the needs, goals and means of touch.

5.10 Thematic Learning Tasks

5.10.1 Reflection Activities

1. Recall the most recent encounter and touching situation with the client. Reflect on this event using the following questions:
   - How did you touch the client? What were your other bodily and sensory gestures and with what kind of tone did you speak to them? Did you touch the client mindfully 'being present' or routinely and mechanically?
   - Can you describe in detail what you experienced in that situation: how did you feel, what kind of affects did you experience?

- Did you experience the touch rewarding and pleasant or was it somehow unpleasant or difficult for you?
- How did you possibly verbalise your touching to the client?
- If you would repeat the encounter, what would you do differently in a similar situation after reading this chapter?

2. Discuss the following questions with your colleagues or peers about your work community:
   - What is the basic mission or task of your organisation and work unit?
   - What kind of values is your organisation officially committed to and how are they embodied in the ways of touching the clients?
   - Are there written or otherwise known rules or guidelines in your organisation about how to touch the client? If not, could it be necessary to formulate them and what kind of principles should there be expressed explicitly?
   - Consider together what kind of touch culture prevails in your organisation and how beneficial touch practices can be promoted in your work community

3. Think about a conflict situation (a real or potential one) with a client where you should use protective, controlling or distancing touch
   - How do you anticipate such a situation and can you somehow prevent it in advance?
   - How do you use touch to protect yourself and others but at the same time treat the client with dignity?
   - Describe what kind of affective or embodied skills you rely on managing the situation

4. Think about what new insights and learnings this chapter has provided to you:
   - What kind of skills and competences do you already hold in terms of embodied ethics regarding your touch practices that you were not aware of before?
   - What weaknesses or limitations have you found in your touch practices that you could develop further?
   - What kind of support and from whom would you need to further develop your skills?

5.10.2 Fieldwork

Embodied ethics as everyday relational practices are difficult to put into words. Therefore, new vocabularies are needed to capture tacit meanings and sensations carried out in this mostly nonverbal bodily interaction. You can advance this verbalisation by conducting a little field work. Choose somebody from your close circle (friends, relatives, colleagues, etc.) to interview them about their experiences as being a client in some sort of 'service' sector (health care, education, social work, fitness, massage, etc.) Examine their answers from the perspective of embodied ethics. Tell them that the interview is related to your studies and this textbook. You can take notes about the interview or ask the interviewee for consent to record the interview. Now, ask them to describe two concrete touching events with the professional when the experience was pleasant and when it was unpleasant. The following questions help you to conduct your interview:

- When and what kind of circumstances did this tactile encounter take place?
- How did the professional touch? Please, try to describe as accurately as possible the nature of the skin contact, for example, a hard grip, a sharp poke, a soothing caress, a light press.
- How would you describe the atmosphere in the situation?
- Why did you possibly feel that the touch was ethically appropriate, for example, compassionate, benevolent or comforting in this situation? Or was it alternatively unethical towards you, for example, insulting, belittling or arrogant?
- Did you have any expectations or special wishes regarding the professional's touch?
- How do you reckon professional touch? What kind of advice, wish or instruction would you like to convey to the professionals?

5.10.3 Case Study

Turn back those two cases introduced in the Sect. 5.9 Box 5.3. (A boisterous child in a day care group) and Box 5.4. (A violent dementia patient in long-term residential care). Read these two cases again and consider the questions in the boxes. Also at the end, answer the following two questions:

- Do you think the professionals' solutions for the situations were ethically sustainable? If yes, in what ways and if not, why is that?
- How would you solve those situations?

References

Alexander, S. (2001). Moral panic in New Zealand: Teachers touching children. In A. Jones (Ed.), *Touchy subject: Teachers touching children* (pp. 87–97). University of Otago Press.
Altintas, E., El Haj, M., Boudoukha, A.-H., Olivier, C., Lizio, A., Luyat, M., & Gallouj, K. (2022). Emotional exhaustion and fear of COVID-19 in geriatric facilities during the COVID-19 pandemic. *PMC International Journal of Geriatric Psychiatry, 37*(8), 10. https://onlinelibrary.wiley.com/doi/epdf/10.1002/gps.5781
Aristotle. (1926). *Nicomachean ethics* (H. Rackham, Trans.). Loeb Classical Library 73. Harvard University Press. https://www.loebclassics.com/view/LCL073/1926/volume.xml
Beauchamp, T. L., & Childress, J. F. (2013 [1985]). *The principles of biomedical ethics* (7th ed.). Oxford University Press.
Benner, P. (2004). Relational ethics of comfort, touch and solace – Endangered arts? *American Joint Committee on Cancer, 13*(4), 346–349.
Bergen, R. (2020). Fear around hugging, touching could be long-term consequence of COVID-19 pandemic, psychologists say. *CBC News,* Apr 27, 2020. https://www.cbc.ca/news/canada/manitoba/covid-19-touch-phobia-manitoba-1.5542899

Bergo, B. (2019). Emmanuel Levinas. *The Stanford encyclopedia of philosophy* (Fall 2019 Edition). In E. N. Zalta (Ed.). https://plato.stanford.edu/archives/fall2019/entries/levinas/

BLM. https://blacklivesmatter.com/transparency/

Bochatay, N. (2018). Individual and collective strategies in nurses' struggle for professional identity. *Health Sociology Review, 27*(3). https://doi.org/10.1080/14461242.2018.1469096

Bonitz, V. (2008). Use of physical touch in the "talking cure": A journey to the outskirts of psychotherapy. *Psychotherapy: Theory/Research/Practice/Training, 45*(2), 391–404.

Brandstetter, G., Egert, G., & Zubarik, S. (2013). *Touching and being touched: Kinesthesia and empathy in dance and movement.* Walter de Gruyter.

Buber, M. (1993). *I and thou.* Authorised translation of Ich und Du (R. G. Smith, Trans.). Continuum.

Bylund-Grenklo, T., Werkander-Harstäde, C., Sandgren, A., Benzein, E., & Östlund, U. (2019). Dignity in life and care: The perspectives of Swedish patients in a palliative care context. *International Journal of Palliative Nursing, 25*(4). https://doi.org/10.12968/ijpn.2019.25.4.193

Bynum, J. P. W., Barre, L., Reed, C., & Passow, H. (2014). Participation of very old adults in healthcare decisions. *Medical Decision Making, 34*(2), 216–230. https://doi.org/10.1177/0272989X13508008

Campanella, T. J. (2000). Eden by wire: Webcameras and the telepresent landscape. In K. Goldberg (Ed.), *The robot in the garden: Telerobotics and telepistomology in the age of the Internet* (pp. 22–45). MIT Press.

Duncan, J. (1999). New Zealand kindergarten teachers and sexual abuse protection policies. *Teaching and Teacher Education, 15*(3), 243–252.

Edgoose, J. Y. C., & Edgoose, J. M. (2017). Finding hope in the face-to-face. *Annals of Family Medicine, 15*(3), 272–274. https://www.annfammed.org/content/annalsfm/15/3/272.full.pdf

Elbqry, M. G., Elmansy, F. M., Elsayed, A. E., Mansour, B., Tantawy, A., Eldin, M. B., & Sayed, H. H. (2021). Effect of COVID-19 stressors on healthcare workers' performance and attitude at Suez Canal university hospitals. *Middle East Current Psychiatry, 28*(4). https://www.ncbi.nlm.nih.gov/pmc/articles/PMC7835443/pdf/43045_2021_Article_84.pdf

Fernandez, R., Lord, H., Halcomb, E., Moxham, L., Middleton, R., Alananzeh, I., & Ellwood, L. (2020). Implications for COVID-19: A systematic review of nurses' experiences of working in acute care hospital settings during a respiratory pandemic. *International Journal of Nursing Studies, 111.* https://doi.org/10.1016/j.ijnurstu.2020.103637

Fischhoff, B., & Barnato, A. E. (2019). Value awareness: A new goal for end-of-life decision making. *MDM Policy & Practice, 4*(1), 1–10. https://doi.org/10.1177/2381468318817523

Fitzgerald, A. (2020). Professional identity: A concept analysis. *Nursing Forum, 55*(3), 447–472. https://doi.org/10.1111/nuf.12450

Foster, S. (2010). *Choreographing empathy. Kinesthesia in performance.* Routledge.

Grigorovich, A., & Kontos, P. (2019). A critical realist exploration of the vulnerability of staff to sexual harassment in residential long-term care. *Social Science & Medicine, 238.* https://doi.org/10.1016/j.socscimed.2019.112356

Guindon, M., Packard, R., & Charron, N. (2017). The ethics of touch in the helping relationships. In M. Rovers, J. Malette, & M. Guirguis-Younger (Eds.), *Touch in the helping professions: Research, practice and ethics* (pp. 213–236). University of Ottawa Press. http://www.jstor.org/stable/j.ctv5vdcvd.16

Guo, Q., & Jacelon, C. S. (2014). An integrative review of dignity in end-of-life care. *Palliative Medicine, 28*(7), 931–940. https://doi.org/10.1177/0269216314528399

Haahr, A., Norlyk, A., Martinsen, B., & Dreyer, P. (2020). Nurses experiences of ethical dilemmas: A review. *Nursing Ethics, 27*(1), 258–272. https://doi.org/10.1177/0969733019832941

Haho, A. (2017). Palliatiivisen vaiheen syöpäpotilaiden eksistentiaalinen kärsimys [Existential suffering of cancer patients in palliative care]. *Lääkärilehti, 72*(33), 1704–1714. https://www.laakarilehti.fi/tieteessa/alkuperaistutkimukset/palliatiivisen-vaiheen-syopapotilaiden-eksistentiaalinen-karsimys/

Haho, A. (2020). *Mitä kärsimys opettaa elämästä? [What suffering teaches about life?].* Tuuma.

Hamrick, A. B. (2014). A case study of moral distress. *Journal of Hospice & Palliative Care, 16*(8), 457–463.

Hamrick, A. B., & Blackhall, L. J. (2007). Nurse-physician perspectives on the care of dying patients in intensive care units: Collaboration, moral distress, and ethical climate. *Critical Care Medicine, 25*(2), 422–429.
Hancock, P. (2009). Management and colonization in everyday life. In P. Hancock & M. Tyler (Eds.), *The Management of everyday life* (pp. 1–20). Palgrave.
Hanna, D. R. (2004). Moral distress: The state of the science. *Research and Theory for Nursing Practice, 18*(1), 73–93. https://pubmed.ncbi.nlm.nih.gov/15083663/
Hännikäinen, M. (2018). Values of well-being and togetherness in the early childhood education of younger children. In E. Johansson & J. Einarsdottir (Eds.), *Values in early childhood education. Citizenship for tomorrow* (pp. 147–162). Routledge.
Hansson, S. O., & Fröding, B. (2021). Ethical conflicts in patient-centred care. *Clinical Ethics, 16*(2), 55–66. https://doi.org/10.1177/1477750920962356
Harrison, C., Jones, R. S. P., & Huws, J. C. (2012). "We're people who don't touch": Exploring clinical psychologists' perspectives on their use of touch in therapy. *Counselling Psychology Quarterly, 25*(3), 277–287.
Hemati, Z., Ashouri, E., Bakhshian, M. A., Pourfarzad, Z., Shirani, F., Safazadeh, S., Ziyaei, M., Varzeshnejad, M., Hashemi, M., & Taleghani, F. (2016). Dying with dignity: A concept analysis. *Journal of Clinical Nursing, 25*(9–10), 1218–1228. https://doi.org/10.1111/jocn.13143
Hockey, J., & Allen-Collinson, J. (2009). The sensorium at work: The sensory phenomenology of the working body. *The Sociological Review, 57*(2), 217–239.
Holopainen, G., Kasen, A., & Nyström, L. (2014). The space of togetherness – A caring encounter. *Scandinavian Journal of Caring Sciences, 28*(1), 186–192.
Horton, J. A., Clance, P. R., Sterk-Elifson, C., & Emshoff, J. (1995). Touch in psychotherapy: A survey of patients' experiences. *Psychotherapy: Theory/Research/Practice/Training, 32*, 443–457.
Hunter, M., & Struve, J. (1998). *The ethical use of touch in psychotherapy*. Sage.
Hursthouse, R., & Pettigrove, G. (2018). Virtue ethics. In E. N. Zalta (Ed.), *The Stanford encyclopedia of philosophy* (Winter 2018 Edition). https://plato.stanford.edu/archives/win2018/entries/ethics-virtue/
ICN, International Council of Nurses. (2022). *The ICN code of ethics for nurses*. https://www.icn.ch/system/files/2021-10/ICN_Code-of-Ethics_EN_Web_0.pdf
ICOEE. (2022). *International code of ethics for educators*. https://static1.squarespace.com/static/572284eec2ea513dc4d683df/t/5bbcbe0d7817f74d89c7ae0f/1539096078523/ICOEE.pdf
Imes, S. (1998). Long-term clients' experience of touch in Gestalt therapy. In E. W. L. Smith, P. R. Clance, & S. Imes (Eds.), *Touch in psychotherapy: Theory, research, and practice* (pp. 170–200). The Guilford Press.
Jameton, A. (1984). *Nursing practice: The ethical issues*. Englewood Cliffs.
Johnson, C. (2020). *Teaching to the test: How schools discourage phronesis*. Routledge.
Johnston, S. H., & Farber, B. A. (1996). The maintenance of boundaries in psychotherapeutic practice. *Psychotherapy, 33*, 391–402.
Kahsay, W. G., Negarandeh, R., Nayeri, N. D., & Hasanpour, N. (2020). Sexual harassment against female nurses: A systematic review. *BioMed Central Nursing, 19*, 58. https://doi.org/10.1186/s12912-020-00450-w
Kant, I. (2003). *Critique of pure reason. Norman Kemp Smith's translation*. Palgrave Macmillan.
Karlsson, M., Karlsson, C., da Silva, B. A., Berggren, I., & Söderlund, M. (2013). Community nurses' experiences of ethical problems in end-of-life care in the patient's own home. *Scandinavian Journal of Caring Sciences, 27*(4), 831–838. https://doi.org/10.1111/j.1471-6712.2012.0108
Keränen, V. (2022). *Moniulotteinen kosketus päiväkodin suhteissa: Kertomuksia varhaiskasvatuksen arjesta* [Multisided touch in preschools' relations – Stories from the everyday life of early childhood education and care]. University of Oulu.
Kinnunen, T., Parviainen, J., Haho, A., & Jolkkonen, M. (2019). *Ammatillinen kosketus. Kuinka tunnetyötä tehdään* [Professional touch. Affective work in practice]. Kirjapaja.
Kröger, T., Puthenparambil, J. M., & Aerschot, L. V. (2019). Care poverty: Unmet care needs in a Nordic welfare state. *International Journal of Care and Caring, 3*(4), 485–500. https://doi.org/10.1332/239788219X15641291564296

Küpers, W. (2012). Inter-communicating – Phenomenological perspectives on embodied communication and con-textuality in organization. *Journal for Communication and Culture, 2*(2), 114–138.

Küpers, W. (2015). Embodied responsive ethical practice. The contribution of Merleau-Ponty for a corporeal ethics in organisations. *Electronic Journal of Business Ethics and Organization Studies, 20*(1), 30–45. Retrieved from http://ejbo.jyu.fi

Ladkin, D. (2015). *Mastering the ethical dimension of organizations. A self-reflective guide to developing ethical astuteness.* Edward Elgar Pub.

Levinas, E. (1985). *Ethics and infinity: Conversations with Philippe Nemo.* Duquesne University Press. (Original work Ethique et infini: Dialogues avec Philippe Nemo published in 1982).

Maiden, J., Georges, J. M., & Connelly, C. D. (2011). Moral distress, compassion fatigue, and perceptions about medication errors in certified critical care nurses. *Dimensions of Critical Care Nursing, 30*(6), 339–345. https://doi.org/10.1097/DCC.0b013e31822fab2a. PMID: 21983510.

Manning, E. (2007). *Politics of touch: Sense, movement, sovereignty.* University of Minnesota Press.

McDowell, J. (1998). *Mind, value, and reality.* Harvard University Press.

Merleau-Ponty, M. (1968). *The visible and the invisible: Followed by working notes* (C. Lefort, Ed. & A. Lingis, Trans.). Northwestern University Press.

Merleau-Ponty, M. (1989 [1962]). *The phenomenology of perception* (C. Smith, Trans.). Routledge. (Original work Phénoménologie de la perception published in 1945).

Milliken, A. (2018). Ethical awareness: What it is and why it matters? *The Online Journal of Issues in Nursing, 23*(1). https://doi.org/10.3912/OJIN.Vol23No01Man01

Mo, S., & Shi, J. (2021). The psychological consequences of the COVID-19 on residents and staff in nursing homes. *Public Health Emergency Collection, 6*(4), 254–259. https://doi.org/10.1093/workar/waaa021

Morgan, M. L. (2007). *Discovering Levinas.* Cambridge University Press. https://doi.org/10.1017/CBO9780511805240

Nielsen, M. B. D., Kjær, S., Aldrich, P. T., Madsen, I. E. H., Friborg, M.-K., Rugulies, R., & Folker, A. P. (2017). Sexual harassment in care work – Dilemmas and consequences: A qualitative investigation. *International Journal of Nursing Studies, 70,* 122–130. https://www.sciencedirect.com/science/article/abs/pii/S0020748917300548?via%3Dihub

Nordtug, E. (2015). Levinas's ethics as a basics of healthcare – Challenges and dilemmas. *Nursing Philosophy, 16*(1), 51–63. https://doi.org/10.1111/nup.12072

Norris, D. M., Gutheil, T. G., & Strasburger, L. H. (2003). This couldn't happen to me: Boundary problems and sexual misconduct in the psychotherapy relationship. *Psychiatric Services, 54*(4), 517–522.

Palukka, H., Haapakorpi, A., Auvinen, P., & Parviainen, J. (2021). Outlining the role of experiential expertise in professional work in health care service co-production. *International Journal of Qualitative Studies on Health and Well-Being, 16*(1), 1–9. https://www.tandfonline.com/doi/epdf/10.1080/17482631.2021.1954744?needAccess=true&role=button

Papastavrou, E., & Suhonen, R. (2021). *Impacts of rationing and missed nursing care: Challenges and solutions.* Springer Nature. https://dokumen.pub/impacts-of-rationing-and-missed-nursing-care-challenges-and-solutions-1nbsped-9783030710729-9783030710736.html

Parviainen, J. (2003). Kinaesthetic empathy. *Dialogue and Universalism, 8*(11–12), 154–165.

Phelan, J. E. (2009). Exploring the use of touch in the psychotherapeutic setting: A phenomenological review. *Psychotherapy: Theory/Research/Practice/Training, 46*(1), 97–111. https://doi.org/10.1037/a0014751

Puroila, A.-M., & Haho, A. (2017). Moral functioning: Navigating the messy landscape of values in Finnish preschools. *Scandinavian Journal of Educational Research, 61*(5), 540–554. https://doi.org/10.1080/00313831.2016.1172499

Puroila, A.-M., Estola, E., Juutinen, J., & Viljamaa, E. (2018). Armchair pedagogy: Embodying caring values in a preschool context. In E. Johansson & J. Einarsdottir (Eds.), *Values in early childhood: Citizenship for tomorrow.* Routledge. http://jultika.oulu.fi/files/nbnfi-fe2018080733466.pdf

Pype, P., Pype, K., Rowlands, A., George, R., & Devisch, I. (2021). COVID-19 and touch in medical encounters. *Patient Education and Counseling, 104*(3), 464–466. https://doi.org/10.1016/j.pec.2020.10.023

Rónay, Z. (2019). Respect for human dignity as a framework and subject of education in the light of present challenges. In *Education applications & developments IV* (Advances in education and educational trends series) (pp. 183–191). In Science Press.

Rushton, C. H., Batcheller, J., Schroeder, K., & Donohue, P. (2015). Burnout and resilience among nurses practicing in high-intensity settings. *American Journal of Critical Care, 24*(5), 412–420. https://doi.org/10.4037/ajcc2015291. PMID: 26330434.

Sandgren, A., Axelsson, L., Bylund-Grenklo, T., & Benzein, S. (2020). Family members' expressions of dignity in palliative care: A qualitative study. *Scandinavian Journal of Caring Sciences, 35*(3), 937–944. https://doi.org/10.1111/scs.12913

Sayers, K. L., & de Vries, K. (2008). A concept development of 'being sensitive' in nursing. *Nursing Ethics, 15*(3), 289–303. https://doi.org/10.1177/0969733007088355

Shaukat, N., Ali, D. M., & Razzak, J. (2020). Physical and mental health impacts of COVID-19 on healthcare workers: A scoping review. *International Journal of Emergency Medicine, 13*(1), 40. https://intjem.biomedcentral.com/articles/10.1186/s12245-020-00299-5

Sihto, T., & Aerschot, L. V. (2021). Care poverty within the home space: Exploring the emotional experiences of unmet care needs. *Frontiers of Sociology, 29.* https://doi.org/10.3389/fsoc.2021.637799

Singer, P. (2011). *Practical ethics* (3rd ed.). Cambridge University Press.

Sipman, G., Thölke, J., Martens, R., & McKenney, S. (2019). The role of intuition in pedagogical tact: Educator views. *British Educational Research Journal, 45*(6), 1186–1202. https://doi.org/10.1002/berj.3557

Stein, E. (1989). *On the problem of empathy* (W. Stein, Trans.). Kluwer. (Original book Zum Problem der Einfühlung published in 1917).

Stenbock-Hult, B., & Sarvimäki, A. (2011). The meaning of vulnerability to nurses caring for older people. *Nursing Ethics, 18*(1), 31–41.

Stover, F. M., & Carlson, F. M. (2006). *Essential touch: Meeting the needs of young children.* National Association for the Education of Young Children.

Styhre, A. (2004). The (re)embodied organization: Four perspectives on the body in organizations. *Human Resource Development International, 7*(1), 101–116. https://doi.org/10.1080/1367886032000150578

Suarez, V., & McGrath, J. (2022). *Teacher professional identity: How to develop and support it in times of change* (OECD education working papers, no. 267). OECD Publishing. https://doi.org/10.1787/b19f5af7-en

Suhonen, R., & Vaarto-Rajalin, H. (2021). Ikääntyneen ihmisen yksilöllisyyden huomioiminen hoitotyössä – osa toteutumatta jäänyttä hoitotyötä? [Taking into account the individuality of elderly people in nursing work – Part of the unfulfilled nursing work]. *Tutkiva Hoitotyö, 19*(3), 40–42. https://urn.fi/URN:NBN:fi-fe202201148509

Tiemersma, D. (1987). Ontology and ethics in the foundation of medicine and the relevance of Levina's view. *Theoretical Medicine and Bioethics, 8*(2), 127–133.

Tistad, M., Tham, K., von Koch, L., & Ytterberg, C. (2012). Unfulfilled rehabilitation needs and dissatisfaction with care 12 months after a stroke: An explorative observational study. *BMC Neurology, 12*(1), 40. https://bmcneurol.biomedcentral.com/articles/10.1186/1471-2377-12-40

Warnecke, T. (2011). Stirring the depths: Transference, countertransference and touch. *Body, Movement and Dance in Psychotherapy, 6*(3), 233–243.

Westland, G. (2011). Physical touch in psychotherapy: Why are we not touching more? *Body, Movement and Dance in Psychotherapy, 6*(1), 17–29.

Weston, J. (1996). *Directing actors. Creating memorable performances for film and television.* M. Wiese Productions.

WHO Code of Ethics. (2022). *World Health Organization.* https://cdn.who.int/media/docs/default-source/documents/ethics/code-of-ethics-pamphlet-en.pdf?sfvrsn=20dd5e7e_3

Wiggins, D. (1998). *Needs, values, truth: Essays in the philosophy of value.* Oxford University Press.

WMA. (2022). *The WMA International Code of Medical Ethics.* https://www.wma.net/wp-content/uploads/2006/09/International-Code-of-Medical-Ethics-2006.pdf
YouGov. (2020). *Eurotrack survey results on sexual harassment.* https://docs.cdn.yougov.com/qepiqi9xaf/YouGov%20Sexual%20harassment.pdf
Zagzebski, L. (1996). *Virtues of the mind: An inquiry into the nature of virtue and the ethical foundations of knowledge.* Cambridge University Press.
Zur, O. (2007). Boundaries in psychotherapy: Ethical and clinical explorations. *American Psychological Association.* https://doi.org/10.1037/11563-000

Further Reading

Aumiller, R. (Ed.). (2021). *A touch of doubt: On haptic scepticism.* Walter de Gruyter.
Ben-Shahar, A. R. (2018). *Touching the relational edge: Body psychotherapy.* Routledge.
Galton, G. (2018). *Touch papers: Dialogues on touch in the psychoanalytic space.* Routledge.
Rovers, M., Malette, J., & Guirguis-Younger, M. (Eds.). (2017). *Touch in the helping professions: Research, practice and ethics.* University of Ottawa Press.
Novak, E. (2022). *Physical touch in psychoanalytic psychotherapy: Transforming trauma through embodied practice.* Routledge.
Todd, S. (2023). *The touch of the present: Educational encounters, aesthetics, and the politics of the senses.* State University of New York Press.

Conclusion: Scenarios and Curriculums of Professional Touch

6

Abstract

The last chapter summarises the book's main points. We highlight the importance of a professional's ethical and socio-cultural competence on touch because even virtual services do not remove the professional's responsibility to encounter clients as living embodied subjects. Additionally, we take a look into the future: how we expect professional touch cultures in client work to develop and what means are available, for example, through socialisation or education to influence touch cultures. We consider different scenarios of touch cultures, and we end by discussing the central role of education in the development of professionals' touch skills. We estimate that in the future, professionals will be increasingly required not only to use technology smoothly, but also to soften the client's experience of being touched with 'cold' technologies and materials or of feeling like an outsider while the professional interacts with technological devices.

6.1 Professional Touch in a Nutshell

In this book, we have stressed three main features of professional touch: touch as professional know-how; touch as a socially learnt practice; touch as a form of embodied ethics in which the client's body is touched mindfully but not in too personal or intimate a manner. To understand professional know-how, we outlined the different functions of professional touch and familiarised the reader with the various intentions or aims professionals may have when they use touch as their working tool. We drew distinctions between (1) connecting touch, (2) procedural touch, (3) assisting and guiding touch, (4) exploratory touch, (5) caring and comforting touch, (6) therapeutic touch, and (7) protective and controlling touch. The identification of these dimensions of the use of touch as a tool in client work can benefit many professionals, helping them not only to grasp the specific nature of their work but also to understand how specific styles of touching contribute to their professional identity and public role.

Throughout the book, we have emphasised that social and technological environments, such as cultural features or digitalisation, affect the ways in which the interaction between professional and client takes shape. Professional touch practices have been patterned in historical, ideological, economic, material and social conditions that comprise comprehensive skinscapes. Therefore, one cannot understand or even perform tactile encounters in client work without considering the cultural factors that are always present in those encounters: the meanings of touch become understandable in cultural contexts—although on the other hand, touch provides a universal communication channel that extends beyond languages and cultures. We illustrated how professional touch styles develop as outcomes of primary and secondary socialisation processes that inherently provide different capacities and affective registers for tactile communication at work. We also stressed that becoming conscious of one's own attachment style, adult tactile relations and culturally adopted manners (such as gendered norms of touch) can enable one to use touch in more versatile and culturally sensitive ways. Similarly, the mechanical tools, instruments and digital technologies used by professionals both enhance and hinder their ability to develop physical contact with clients. We introduced a novel approach that we called 'technology-mediated touch' to show how technological tools shape tactile interactions between professionals and clients.

We formulated the notion of embodied ethics in order to understand more profoundly how professionals can be present with, encounter or act with their clients in fair and ethically sustainable ways, taking into account the many factors that may limit their tactile interactions. Normative ethics considers the needs of the individual client but rests above all on universal human rights, legal guidelines and professional knowledge about human well-being. We underlined the reciprocity of touch, which also influences professional work, sometimes in unpredictable ways. Consequently, the importance of a professional's ethical competence with regard to decision-making, procedures and value awareness must not be underestimated, because these factors are directly reflected and concretely embodied in client encounters and reciprocal touch. For this reason, it is also important to consider the moral distress caused to professionals by touch.

In what follows, we take a look into the future: how we expect professional touch cultures in client work to develop, and what means are available (e.g. through socialisation or education) to influence touch cultures. We consider different scenarios of touch cultures, and we end by discussing the central role of education in the development of professionals' touch skills.

6.2 Alternative Scenarios for the Future of Professional Touch

Professional touch in client encounters is facing many threats and challenges. As we have stated, the global pandemic (infection control by social distancing), sexual harassment (touching in inappropriate ways, and fear of touching in inappropriate

6.2 Alternative Scenarios for the Future of Professional Touch

ways) and service digitisation in high-tech societies have already changed the forms of tactile interaction in client work in many sectors. In addition, loneliness, social isolation and the rise of living alone—which are related to the emphasis on individuality and independence, especially in Western societies—inevitably affect how healthcare and education services are designed, for example, and the role touch plays in those services. Thus, possible scenarios for touch cultures in the future may be influenced not only by factors that change cultures slowly but also, as we have seen, by rapid, even radical changes that can immediately affect tactile interactions between professionals and clients. In the light of the slow and rapid changes that have already taken place, we have suggested that modern societies are partially developing in touch-deprived or even touch-phobic directions. There is no single reason for this phenomenon: digitisation or the pandemic alone are not enough to explain it. We can speculate as to whether modern people actively prefer to deal with the authorities remotely or through a digital system rather than face to face, or whether digital systems are being implemented in services with the result that face-to-face services are no longer available. Does the root cause lie in technological and social reforms that push changes in people's behaviour? Or vice versa, do changes in people's behaviour and values generate social and technological reforms? Perhaps the correct answer is a combination of both.

We can roughly divide future scenarios into those where touching and physical interactions between clients and professionals decrease even further, and those where the touch culture is consciously cultivated in light of various interventions, education and research. We draw attention to concerns about the decrease in touch contacts due to digitalisation, fears and prohibitions related to touch, the underestimation of the importance of skin contact, and the increase of touch depression among some citizen groups. We are also concerned about the development of inequality in society, which relates to touch on at least two levels: (1) inequalities in emotional or affective resources acquired during childhood and in later intimate relations (2) inequalities in touch-based services, whereby touch becomes a privilege of wealthy clients, while poor people have to settle for mechanised and automatic services. We want to address the fact that individuals have different primary care backgrounds, and this in itself creates affective inequalities in society. This means that in all client work environments, there are individuals—both clients and professionals—whose opportunities and capacities to benefit from caring touch are less favourable compared with those who have experienced touch as a positive resource in their lives. We are concerned about how this inequality might be better met in client work, because a well-considered professional touch obviously has tremendous potential to compensate less fortunate clients and professionals for their lack of touch-related affective capital, as many real-life examples presented in this book have demonstrated.

The development of economic inequality in society also affects the availability of touch-based services in many ways. Thanks to cuts and savings in the public sector, many face-to-face services may be transformed into digitalised online self-services. According to this scenario, digitalisation will automate the services offered to citizens in such a way that a face-to-face meeting with a professional will be arranged only in special cases. Simply put, if the number of encounters with professionals decreases, the amount of tactile contact also decreases. This lack of services will manifest itself especially in the care of old adults, and at worst will lead to violations of basic human rights. The backdrop to this scenario might be a shortage of employees, problems in meeting the needs of services and clients, a failure to organise the work in effective ways, or other insufficiencies of resources. Touch deprivation in client work also includes mechanised care or care provided by remote connections where the nurse's touch and presence has been eliminated. Unfulfilled care means that the needs of the client, including the need to be seen and touched, remain unrealised. In addition, unfulfilled care seems to have a strong connection with the ethical burden that employees suffer when they encounter their clients' suffering but lack the resources to help them.

Further, many services related to well-being, health, beauty and fitness are accompanied by professional face-to-face guidance and comforting touch, with the potential result that human touch is seen as a luxury. Nonetheless, despite these threatening future scenarios, we want to believe that knowledge and understanding of the positive and rewarding effects of touch—not only for the client, but also for professionals themselves—will spread among service providers in basic or public services. When a touch evokes a positive affect in both parties, this reciprocity can be understood as a bond that enhances trust and cohesion between them.

We have taught touch skills and ethics to professionals, many of whom have told us that they have become more careful about touching, or even try to avoid it altogether, in the wake of child abuse scandals and #Metoo. Prior to the 1980s, no-touch policies in educational settings were uncommon. Since the 1990s, touch has become highly regulated (but not entirely forbidden) between teachers and students, even though the general culture may have become more favourable to caring and loving touches. In line with the other environments discussed in Chap. 3, some conservatories and music schools in Finland today ask parents to complete a permission slip to allow teachers to touch students while teaching them to sing or play an instrument. Although asking for written permission indicates responsibility and a desire to eradicate harmful touch, at the same time it makes touching formal, conditional and subject to licence. Professional work will easily become bureaucratised if most interactions in functional situations require written agreements or informed consent in nurseries, schools and other client work institutions and organisations. The request for written permission may itself also arouse the suspicion of potentially inappropriate or dangerous situations. By being cautious and distant, teachers implicitly show children that they as adults cannot be trusted because they cannot be alone in proximity with a child (Alexander, 2001). Not all such fears are related to the risk of accusations of sexual harassment; some stem from the professional's own background, as we have stated. In any case, such fears can prevent the professional from developing the skill to use touch in versatile ways in different work tasks, which is harmful not only to the professional themselves but above all to their clients.

The digitisation of services, combined with the general decrease of touching between strangers (including professionals and clients), can lead to a situation where touch is seen as belonging exclusively to intimate or personal relationships among family members or other loved ones. In this scenario, the touch between the professional and the client becomes strictly regulated, and skin contact is associated only with intimate relationships. Using Edward T. Hall's (1963) proxemics and its four distance zones—intimate, personal, social and public zones—it can be argued that touch in this scenario would be related only to the intimate and personal zones, and would not extend to the social zone. If the professional is responsible only for client tasks that they can perform at a distance, touch becomes privatised, and skin contact is allowed only on occasions where just family members, friends, neighbours or loved ones are present. In this (to us) undesirable scenario, touch is understood mainly in terms of the right *not* to be touched. The result is an impoverishment of the touch culture such that physical contact between strangers is considered inherently suspicious and to be avoided, and skin contact in client work is reduced to strictly necessary caring, nursing or other procedures.

Perhaps the worst-case scenario for the future of professional touch is that touching skills will remain highly undervalued. Although touch is considered to be a significant factor in the promotion of human well-being and health, work where touch is used is not appreciated, and touch work is not rewarded at all in terms of salary. Touching is seen only as a necessity or as a self-evident feature of work tasks, although it is a sensitive skill that requires training. However, if touch is associated with professions that require little education and yield low incomes, it will continue to confer low status in the labour market, in which case highly educated professionals will maintain physical distance from their clients ever more carefully, albeit often unconsciously. The overspecialisation of professions, whereby different professions focus on highly specific problems, can easily lead to the impoverishment of holistic client encounters. Thus, for example, an ear, nose and throat specialist is not allowed to touch the patient, because the duty of touching falls to the practical nurse.

Although we have pinpointed some negative consequences of the #Metoo movement for touch cultures, it has certainly brought many positive effects including, for a growing number of professionals and industry bodies, a renewed attention and moral sensitivity to tactile interaction with clients. Similarly, the global COVID-19 crisis has sharpened the meanings of touch, since people have noticed how important—although often taken for granted—tactile contact is in mundane situations, and how crucial it is for human well-being. In many organisations, managers and professionals have discovered how difficult it is to create working conditions and facilities for professionals where client contact is minimised. As a result, many professionals feel the need to develop their own touch skills and to deepen their understanding of ethical guidance concerning the use of touch at work. This development opens up a positive new scenario where the focus is on increasing the appreciation of touch through research and learning. Table 6.1 lists four sets of agents that can have a substantial impact on the development of tactile interactions: (1) researchers and educators, (2) work organisations, (3) professionals and (4) clients. We recommend that readers pay special attention to the actions and policies that are necessary to bring about the positive, versatile and productive usage of touch in professional practices.

Table 6.1 Prerequisites for the realisation of a positive touch scenario

Agent	Actions needed
Researchers and educators	Funding private and public research programmes to develop touch research, especially in the humanities and social sciences Increasing touch education at all educational levels, especially adult education Developing pedagogy and materials to teach professional touch in theory and practice
Work organisations	Clearly stating the role of tactile interaction in the organisation's basic mission, ethics and values Committing to the principle that professional touch is essential for the well-being of clients and employees Adjusting time scales for encounters with clients Providing appropriate salaries to recognise the application of touch skills in work tasks Organising training in touch skills and embodied ethics Providing peer support and support from supervisors Publicly advocating the importance of touch as part of good and effective client work

Professionals	Knowledge:
	  Acquiring multidisciplinary theoretical and evidence-based knowledge about the meanings and effects of touch
	  Studying professional ethics and its applications in practical work
	  Acquiring multifaceted knowledge about interaction skills and culturally sensitive touch practices
	  Identifying vulnerable client groups who are not able to express their wishes and needs for touch but would potentially benefit from it the most, such as children, people with developmental disabilities or memory impairments, psychiatric patients and hospice patients
	Stance and attitude:
	  Appreciating the skills of professional touch as part of good and effective client work, understanding them as a strong indication of professional competence
	  Understanding that the values of occupational groups and organisations are conveyed through touch practices
	  Reflecting on one's own background related to experiences of touch and how it might resonate in tactile client encounters
	  Adopting the idea that professional touch is fundamentally an equal right but needs attuning to the client's individual needs
	  Consciously processing the principles of ethically sustainable touch
	Concrete touch skills:
	  Practising sensitivity to identify clients' needs for tactile and other sensory interactions
	  Developing the skill to use touch for different functions, and encouraging other professionals to do likewise
	  Acknowledging clients' right to access information, and always explaining to them in advance how and why they are going to be touched
	  Discussing with the client their attitudes, wishes and expectations regarding touch
	  Supporting clients to share the fears and difficult past experiences of touch, if they express a need to do so
	  Justifying touch in relation to legally based professional goals
	  Strengthening the human role in triadic touch situations by providing appropriate information and paying attention to the client in other ways, such as by making eye contact or speaking calmly
	  Recognising challenging situations where it is reasonable to withdraw from potentially dangerous touch situations
	  Being able to use controlling touch when necessary in respectful ways

(continued)

Table 6.1 (continued)

Agent	Actions needed
Clients	Setting aside sufficient time for the encounter and necessary procedures
	Acknowledging one's own experiences, memories, wishes and fears related to touch in the past and present
	Expressing one's preferred way to be touched by the professional and letting them know about it
	Respecting the privacy of professionals

6.3 Should Touch Skills Be Added to Organisational Mission Statements and Educational Curriculums?

Touch is a versatile, powerful, delicate and nuanced working tool, and it can be strengthened by means of various educational and training practices. The implementation of touch in organisational work practices in ways that realise its full potential is never cost-free: it requires educational and time resources. However, the benefit the organisation will receive from investing in the development of employees' touch skills can be substantial, since the sensitive use of touch brings significant qualitative content to the interaction and increases the well-being of clients and professionals alike. For this reason, the promotion of touch skills can increase the efficiency and humanity of organisations, which is ultimately cost-effective too: it advances the outcomes of the work in the form of clients' and employees' well-being. Organisations also have the opportunity to help to promote a positive touch culture, not just in the whole working community but even in the whole of society.

In Box 6.1, we present a list we have compiled to summarise the working skills and professional ethics that we think individual employees and organisations need if they wish to meet the criteria for ideal tactile interactions with clients. Box 6.2 summarises why touch skills should be included in educational curriculums in fields where touch is a necessary part of client work. We describe the content and goals this touch education should include to ensure that students attain sufficient skills and knowledge about professional touch. All of the themes in both boxes have been explored in depth in this book.

Systematic training in touch skills as an independent subject is absent from most client work training programmes, including in the sectors where they are most needed, such as education and healthcare. Of course, one-off practical courses in touching skills such as kinaesthetics (Box 2.3) are included as technical measures in some subject areas, such as elder care, ergonomics, rehabilitation, physiotherapy and psychotherapy (e.g. body psychotherapy). As we have stated, the digitalisation of professional operating environments does not remove the need for physical encounters, but rather the opposite: skills in multisensory interaction and intentional touching are even more necessary in technologised work environments. Thus, we propose that training in professional touch skills should be included in official curriculums for social and healthcare professionals, early childhood educators and subject teachers. It is also necessary to add this training to specialist vocational

Box 6.1 Skills and Ethics of Touch Required from Individual Employees and Organisations

Embodied knowledge about touching skills:

- Being able to use various forms of touch (Sect. 2.1)
- Having practical wisdom (phronesis) about touch, that is, skills (e.g. presence, empathy and sensitivity) to face the client in situation-specific ways
- Being able to reflect on negative and positive impacts of touch, for example, learning from one's mistakes
- Being able to manage one's own touch in such a way that the touch will have a beneficial affective impact on the client
- Being aware of how technologies and tools influence client interactions

Knowledge of embodied ethics:

- Understanding the reciprocity and intercorporeality of touch
- Learning to handle the moral dilemmas (e.g. moral distress) that touch can cause in embodied interactions
- Developing organisations in such a way that it becomes possible to realise the conditions for embodied ethics

Skills to apply global and local professional ethical codes in relation to touch:

- Internalising core principles of professional ethics
- Applying local and private declarations of professional ethics into one's own organisation or workplace

Knowledge about the legislation governing professional activities:

- Knowing the rights and responsibilities of clients and employees

Organisational knowledge about the basic mission and the promotion of touch culture:

- Identifying the role of touch in necessary work tasks and interactions, and realising the potential to promote touch skills and develop a touch-friendly culture
- Exploring the attitudinal and experiential atmosphere regarding professional touch
- Establishing basic moral principles to create a safe space for all actors
- Actively collecting evidence-based information about good tactile practices to strengthen professional expertise

Box 6.2 Content and Goals of Touch Education
Practical training:

- Practical training and experimentation in touching under safe conditions with peers
- Practical skills to handle different forms of professional touch (Chap. 2) and use technical tools as part of the interaction (Chap. 4)
- Practising to recognise the harmful and beneficial effects of different intentional touches
- Training to confront aggressive clients
- Training to handle groups of vulnerable clients
- Development of culturally sensitive multisensory interaction skills

Knowledge about professional ethics:

- Basic principles of professional ethics and guidelines
- Normative ethics of touching, that is, when touch must be avoided or is prohibited
- Introduction to embodied ethics and its principles
- Understanding of how professional identity is constructed

Knowledge of touch cultures:

- Socialisation to touch through different attachment styles and affective repertoires (Chap. 3)
- Diversity of touch cultures, skinscapes and meanings of touch
- Gendered and sexualised professional touch
- Organisational cultures
- Collegial reflection on correct touch practices that promote the client's well-being

Knowledge of physiology and the lived body:

- Parasympathetic nervous system
- Oxytocin
- Hapticity
- Kinesthesis

Knowledge about technology-mediated touch:

- Digitalisation and its impact on touching
- Touching in and through technologies

(continued)

> **Box 6.2** (continued)
> - Triadic relationships
> - Emerging technologies and touching
>
> Knowledge about profession-specific clients:
>
> - Newborns, small children, young people, old adults
> - Children and students with special needs
> - People with learning disabilities
> - People with dementia or Alzheimer's disease
> - People with mental health difficulties
> - People with drug or alcohol abuse disorders
> - Marginalised people and other vulnerable clients
>
> Pedagogy of teaching professional touch:
>
> - Developing new methods to train students in practical touching skills and advance theory

qualifications for beauticians, athletics coaches, adult educators and trainers, vocational teachers and special needs teachers. After all, almost all client work necessitates touch skills, if only to create a connection with the client when one greets them, no matter whether one is a salesperson, dressmaker, car dealer, massage therapist, security guard, waiter or concierge.

In the future, professionals will be increasingly required not only to use technology smoothly, but also to soften the client's experience of being touched with 'cold' technologies and materials or of feeling like an outsider while the professional interacts with technological devices. The centrality of social media and virtual services in client interactions does not remove the professional's responsibility to encounter clients through touch when it is to the client's benefit to do so. Quite the contrary: the power of embodied presence and touch will be greater than ever.

References

Alexander, S. (2001). Moral panic in New Zealand: Teachers touching children. In A. Jones (Ed.), *Touchy subject: Teachers touching children* (pp. 87–97). University of Otago Press.

Hall, E. T. (1963). A system for the notation of proxemic behavior. *American Anthropologist, 65*(5), 1003–1026.

Research Material 7

7.1 Quoted Interviews

'Annika', nursing teacher, 19.12.2017 (date of interview)
   'Eila', nursing teacher, 19.12.2017
   'Eero', nurse in home care, 16.12.2016
   'Elma', nurse in geriatric ward, 28.2.2017
   'Emma', nursing student, 21.12.2017
   'Hanna', nurse in geriatric ward, 30.3.2017
   'Hilkka', practical nurse in sheltered home, 21.2.2017
   'Iida', nursing student, 2017
   'Jonna', practical nurse in home care, 15.2.2017
   'Kaisa', practical nurse in long-term care unit, 21.2.2017
   'Liisa', practical nurse in psychogeriatric ward, 12.4.2017
   'Rebekka', practical nurse in geriatric ward, 22.2.2017
   'Reetta', 57-year-old female patient in hospice care unit, 8.4.2015
   'Sami', masseur, 2012
   'Sari', practical nurse in home care, 13.1.2017
   'Seija', physiotherapy teacher, 19.12.2017
   'Seppo', schoolteacher, 2008
   'Sirkka', nurse in geriatric ward, 23.2.2017
   'Sofia', practical nurse in long-term care unit, 24.2.2017
   'Tanja', nursing student, 20.12.2017
   'Tiina', nursing student, 20.12.2017
   'Tyyne', nurse in geriatric ward, 18.3.2018
   'Vilma', practical nurse in geriatric ward, 22.2.2017

7.2 Archive Materials

'Eini', nurse, has written touch biography to the public call titled *Touch in Finland—warmth, trust or fear?* (Finnish Literature Society, period of the call 2011–2012)

'Helka', has written touch biography to the public call titled *Touch in Finland—warmth, trust or fear?* (Finnish Literature Society 2011–2012)

'Laura', has written narrative to the public call titled *That nurse I will not forget* (Finnish Literature Society, year of the call 2000)

'Merja', nurse, has written touch biography to the public call titled *Touch in Finland—warmth, trust or fear?* (Finnish Literature Society 2011–2012)

'Nina', has written narrative to the public call titled *That nurse I will not forget* (Finnish Literature Society 2000)

'Pekka', nurse, has written touch biography to the public call titled *Touch in Finland—warmth, trust or fear?* (Finnish Literature Society, 2011–2012)

Index

Numbers and symbols
#Metoo, 5–8, 93, 96, 143, 145, 172, 184, 185

A
Actor-network theory (ANT), 122
Aestheticisation, 32
Affect, 8, 10–13, 20, 22, 23, 30, 42, 45, 50, 51, 56, 58–61, 65, 66, 72, 77, 82, 85, 100–102, 107, 108, 114, 116, 122, 124, 128, 134, 137, 143, 154, 155, 157, 164, 169, 173, 182–184
Affective repertoire, 23, 57, 71, 75–78, 97, 189
Affective touch, 63, 129
Affective work, 3, 10, 12, 22, 59, 60, 95, 154
African, 80, 89, 90, 95
Age, 3, 12, 14, 20, 39, 66, 72, 81–83, 93, 97, 114, 167
Ageing body, 82
Aggressive behaviours, 35, 133, 170
Aggressive touch, 60
Alcohol abuse disorder, 151, 190
Alternative medicine, 46
Altruism, 147
Alzheimer's disease, 53, 170, 190
Ambivalent attachment style, 73, 75, 76
America/-n, 13, 45, 55, 81, 94–96, 100, 111, 119, 130
Amyotrophic lateral sclerosis, 46
Analogic machine, 117
Anatomical-physiological schema, 45
Anatomy, 40
Andrieu, Bernard, 91, 98, 99
Anglo-Saxon, 81
Animal, 15, 77, 85–89, 102, 122, 127, 129, 131, 132, 153
Anorexic, 49

Anthropologist/anthropology, 14, 16, 33, 74, 79, 85
Anxiety, 6, 40, 43, 60, 64, 73, 77, 87, 94, 113, 133, 136, 151, 164, 165
Arab, 80, 81, 100
Aristotle, 14, 149
Armchair pedagogy, 167
Artefact, 111, 113, 118, 119, 121, 129–131, 153
Arterial cannula, 47
Artificial intelligence (AI)-operated devices, 117
Asian, 80, 89, 100
Assisting touch, 38–40
Athlete, 53, 94, 95
Athletics coach, 3, 38, 172, 190
Atmosphere, 11, 40, 43, 49, 51, 65, 77, 84, 115, 121, 150, 155, 170, 171, 175, 188
Attachment figure, 72–74
Attachment model theory, 73, 74, 76, 77
Attachment style, 23, 71–76, 78, 97, 101, 182, 189
Auditive message, 50
Auditory sensation, 50
Australia, 4, 89
Authentic existence, 156
Automation, 63, 109, 124–129
Autonomy, 85, 122, 129, 146, 147, 157, 162
Avoidance of touch, 5, 7, 60, 82, 154, 173
Avoidant attachment style, 76

B
Baker, Camille, 115, 116
Beauchamp, Tom, 146, 147, 149

Beautician, 3, 8, 9, 34, 41, 49, 57, 60, 117, 123, 130, 190
Beauty industry, services, 12
Beauty salon, 49
Benedict, Ruth, 74
Beneficence, 146, 147
Bioethical principles, 147
Biomechatronic body part, 125
Black Lives Matter, 145
Blind, 116, 117
Blocking tactic, 60
Blood pressure, 36, 41
Blood sample, 36, 41, 48, 97, 120
Bodily extension, 124
Body culture, 79
Body language, 32, 51, 62, 63
Body part, 14, 34, 35, 37, 40, 42, 49, 56, 61, 62, 79, 80, 96, 125
Body posture, 39, 50
Body psychotherapy, 45, 46, 187
Body technique, 79
Body work, 8–13, 21, 29, 31, 64
Bourdieu, Pierre, 117
Bowlby, John, 73
Brazilian, 95
Britain, British, 73, 95
Buber, Martin, 145, 156, 157
Business model, 109

C
Cameroon, 83
Cannula, cannulisation, 47, 120, 121, 123
Care robotics, 3, 128
Caribbean, 99, 100
Caring touch, 7, 15–17, 31, 42, 44, 45, 48, 54, 58, 76–78, 88, 92, 121, 128, 183
Catholic Church, 96
Cavallone, Mauro, 109, 110, 113
Child abuse, 7, 94, 164, 184
Childcare, 23, 71, 72, 74, 75, 90, 94
Childress, James, 146, 147, 149
China, 80
Class, 12, 40, 72, 74, 79, 81–83, 87, 112, 156, 157
Classen, Constance, 14, 56, 78, 79, 87, 89, 91
Collectivism, 80
Comforting touch, 9, 23, 29, 42–45, 48, 60, 89, 102, 103, 123, 181, 184
Companion species, 125
Complementary medicine, 46
Connecting touch, 13, 22, 29, 33–35, 47, 64, 65, 163, 181
Consequentialism, 146

Contact culture, 95
Contact zone, 80
Contamination, 87
Controlling touch, 23, 29, 46–47, 59, 60, 75, 92, 181
Convalescent patient, 46
Co-sleeping, 82
Cosmetologist, 49
COVID-19 pandemic, 4–6, 23, 34, 38, 82, 85, 87, 108–110, 113, 131–133, 137, 145, 164, 172
Critical technology studies, 23, 107
Cross-cultural, 34, 80, 83, 89, 97, 100
Cross-gender, 80, 81, 93
C-Tactile fibres/afferents, 15
Cultural background, 13, 55, 61, 62, 84, 98–101, 151, 156
Cultural competence, 83, 84
Cultural context, 12, 18, 74, 75, 93, 97, 182
Cultural diversity, 83
Cultural habit, 12, 84, 97
Cultural sensitivity, 83, 84, 101
Cultural stereotype, 90, 91
Culture-bound touch, 78–83
Curriculum, 36, 60, 122, 181–190
Cybernetic/-s, 111, 125
Cyborg, 124–129

D
Dance teacher, 38
Day care centres, 94, 170
Deafblind, 173
Deep feeling, 37, 58
Dementia care/patient, 31, 43, 48, 53, 55, 86, 102, 168
Dentist, 31, 120, 123
Deontology, 148
Depression, 43, 133, 158, 165, 183
Descriptive ethics, 19, 148–151, 169
Dialysis machine, 117, 119
Digital bubble, 113, 115
Digital connection, 108–109
Digital devices, 20, 22, 90, 109, 114, 117, 119, 121, 125
Digitalisation, 3, 6, 14, 21, 23, 87, 90, 108–113, 132, 136–138, 143, 145, 182, 183, 187, 189
Digital proxemics, 112–116
Digital space, 113, 114
Dignity, 6, 17, 18, 20, 37, 128, 146, 150, 151, 155, 160–165, 169, 171, 173, 174
Disabled people, 38, 151
Disorganised attachment style, 74, 76

Distress, 5, 74, 144, 162, 165, 168–173, 182, 188
Doctor, 3, 4, 7, 21, 22, 36, 41, 42, 49, 59, 77, 88, 89, 91, 93, 100, 120, 125, 126, 130, 137, 156, 161
Dog, 17, 88, 125, 127
Dreyfus, Hubert, 63, 111, 130
Drug delivery robot, 126
Drug use, 173
Dyadic relationship, 120, 123
Dying, 5, 13, 15, 16, 44, 83, 152, 158, 160–162

E

Early childhood, 2, 20, 23, 31, 54, 56, 71, 72, 80, 99, 100, 144, 155, 156, 163–165, 167, 170, 187
Early childhood education, 31, 80, 100, 163–165
Ear, nose and throat specialists, 31
Eating disorders, 133
Economic
  conditions, 117
  factors, 12, 75
  structures, 90
Ecosystem of devices, 131
Educational institution, 110, 164
Elderly care, 6, 21, 37, 47, 83, 100, 127, 155, 163
Elema, Riekje, 5, 8, 35, 36, 47, 52, 59, 63, 64
Embodied ethics, 12, 19, 23, 143, 149, 152–155, 157, 159, 160, 174, 181, 182, 188, 189
Embodied memory, 60
Emergency care, 36, 41, 47, 59, 83, 92
Emotional exhaustion, 163
Emotional intimacy, 44, 55
Emotional resource, 36, 60
Emotional work, 10, 12, 58, 172
Emotion management, 10, 58
Emotions, 2, 8, 10–12, 14, 15, 17, 30, 43, 56–61, 64, 65, 94, 147, 154, 156, 158, 159, 162, 164, 169–171
Empathy, 2, 19, 42, 54, 58, 123, 128, 155–160, 173, 188
End-of-life care, 53, 158, 160–162
England/English, 80, 100, 172
Estabrooks, Carole A., 31, 32, 60, 80
Ethical codes, 18, 145, 146, 149, 188
Ethical dilemma, 18, 36, 88, 144–145, 169
Ethical theory, 153
Ethnic/ethnicity, 12, 72, 79–81, 83, 88, 97, 102
Ethnography/ethnographic, 49, 53, 65, 82

Etiquette, 34, 65, 78, 96, 97
Europe/-an, 79–81, 87–91, 95
Evidence-based intervention, 152
Evolution, 13, 92
Exoskeleton, 124
Exploratory touch, 23, 29, 41–42, 181
Eye contact, 43, 48, 50, 79, 93, 100, 168

F

Facial expression, 14, 50, 62, 167
Fauci, Anthony, 131
Feeling rules, 10, 12, 32, 55, 58
Female, 7, 14, 32, 58, 81, 89–95, 97, 100, 159, 164, 172
Filipino, 86, 88
Finland, 3, 4, 49, 76, 81, 88, 90, 115, 184
Fitness instructor, 3, 40, 127
Floatation therapy, 130
Four-handed surgical robot, 124, 125
French, 33, 79, 80, 91, 112, 122
Freud, Sigmund, 163

G

Game, 80, 114, 124
Gathering-around technologies, 6, 114, 116
Gendered touch, 13, 72, 81
Genital area, 96
Geriatric nurse, 83, 98
Geriatric ward, 3, 31, 44, 118, 168
Gerontology, 5, 62
Gleeson, Madeline, 4, 31, 34, 35, 38, 42, 47, 57, 62, 93–95, 97
Gloves, 1, 5, 6, 10, 36, 59, 83, 102, 121, 134, 161
Grip, 33, 39, 45, 54, 56, 60–63, 168, 175
Guiding touch, 22, 29, 38–40, 181
Gustatory sensation, 50

H

Habit memory, 63
Habitus, 107, 117, 118, 134
Hairdresser, 17, 34
Hall, Edward T., 79, 80
Handshake, 20, 33, 34, 45, 50, 51, 62, 93, 99, 100, 134
Hands-on healing method, 91
Haptece, 53
Hapteme, 53
Haptic/haptics, 14, 87, 110, 111, 125, 126, 130, 131, 133, 134
Haraway, Donna, 111, 122, 124, 125

Hayles, Katherine, 111, 112
Healing energy, 46
Healthcare chatbots, 110
Healthcare professional, 4, 9, 32, 41, 42, 44, 54, 57, 60, 61, 84, 88, 93, 97, 113, 119, 120, 123, 127, 145, 152, 162, 165, 187
Hedonism, 146
Hermeneutic relation, 119, 123
Hierarchies/hierarchy, 14, 51, 56, 82, 83, 88, 89, 91, 122
Higgins, Agnes, 4, 31, 34, 35, 38, 42, 47, 57, 62, 93–95, 97
High-touch (touch-intensive) work, 20, 83, 90
Hikikomori, 133
Hindu, 93, 96, 97
Historical context, 75
Hochschild, Arlie, 10, 12, 55, 58
Home care, 1–3, 38, 54, 78, 115, 126, 129, 133, 172
Homosexuality, 81, 92, 95
Hospital, 3, 9, 20, 35, 36, 38, 42, 49, 51, 52, 54, 83, 85, 86, 95, 99, 113, 117, 119–121, 123, 124, 126, 132
Hug, 7, 20, 34, 44, 47, 78, 81, 95, 97, 131, 164, 167
Human-computer interaction (HCI), 111, 157
Human-machine interaction, 14, 110, 111, 113
Humanoid robot, 123, 127
Human rights, 18, 23, 38, 143, 160, 169, 182, 184
Hygiene care, 36, 48, 51

I

Ihde, Don, 111, 119, 123, 125, 126, 130
Inanimate being, 125
Incontinence, 2, 37, 78, 166
Individualism, 80
Industrialisation, 87, 90
Inequalities/inequality, 76, 183
Infantilise, 94
Information and communications technologies (ICTs), 109, 110, 113
Information system, 113, 123, 126
Injection, 36, 121, 123
Inorganic prosthesis or implant, 124
Insecure attachment style, 73–75
Instrumental touch, 9, 31, 38, 39, 45, 165
Intelligent device, 129
Intensive care, 36, 92
Intention/-al, 11, 17, 20, 30–32, 34, 36, 37, 43, 44, 47, 49, 51, 52, 65, 76, 78, 112, 122, 123, 134, 151, 154, 157, 163, 171, 172, 181, 187
International recommendations, 144, 145
Intimacy, 5, 15, 44, 55, 73, 92, 118, 131, 149
Intimate hygiene, 1, 37, 38
Intimate zone, 79, 80, 114
Intubation tube, 47
Investigative touch, 9, 41
Inviolability, 37
Ireland, 4, 34, 62

J

Japan/-ese, 80–82, 95, 133
Jewish, 80

K

Kant, Immanuel, 147, 148
Kelly, Martina Ann, 8, 21, 31, 42, 47, 54, 85, 92, 93
Keränen, Virve, 31, 43, 100, 165
Kinaesthesia, 14, 39, 118
Kindergarten, 82
Kinesthetic empathy, 159
Kinetic, 47, 50, 131
Kiss, 13, 34, 65, 81, 95, 97
Korea, 80

L

Lab nurse, 41
Labour market, 90, 166, 185
Laptop, 112, 127
Latour, Bruno, 111, 122
Legal guideline, 19, 23, 61, 143, 182
Legislation, 18, 145, 188
Levinas, Emmanuel, 152, 153, 156
Lifting aid, 129
Lived body, 107, 112, 117, 159, 189
Local anaesthetic, 37
Lockdown, 7, 110, 132, 133
Loneliness, 87, 96, 126, 158, 162, 163, 183
Long-term care unit, 52, 54, 167
Long-term residential care, 171, 175
Love, 10, 14, 15, 20, 44, 56, 100, 162
Loving touch, 44, 58, 184
Lowered self-esteem, 43, 133
Low-touch work, 80, 88, 90
Loyalty, 160
Lupton, Deborah, 117

Index

M
Male, 7, 34, 37, 45, 65, 77, 81, 85, 86, 90–95, 97, 100, 133, 163, 164, 172
Manning, Erin, 10, 47, 155
Manual instrument, 90
Masculinity, 89, 91, 92
Massage, 11, 19, 45, 49, 62, 76, 89, 117, 159, 174, 190
Masseur, 3, 8, 9, 19, 34, 45, 49, 57, 62, 63, 88, 102, 123
Material entity, 112
Materiality, 111, 122
Material objects, 11, 23, 107, 108, 110, 116, 120, 122–124, 129
Material touch, 129–131
Mathematical algorithms, 124
Mauss, Marcel, 79
Mead, Margaret, 74
Mechanical muscle, 124
Mechanical tools, 107, 108, 111, 134, 182
Medical justification, 36
Medical practice/procedure/treatment, 5, 35, 36, 42, 47, 58, 88, 91, 92, 96
Medical specialist/instructor, doctor, 4, 31, 88, 91
Medicine, 16, 31, 46, 49, 89, 91, 124, 126, 138, 147
Memory (sensory), 14
Memory impairment/disorder, 7, 43, 162, 170, 171
Mental condition, 93, 117
Mental health problem, 132
Mental health professional, 163
Mental representation, 156
Merleau-Ponty, Maurice, 111, 112, 116–119, 129, 130, 153, 154
Middle Ages, 81, 87
Middle Eastern, 90
Mirror neurons, 14
Mistreatment, 60
Mobile app, 108
Mobile phone, 112, 114–116, 119, 125
Moral distress, 144, 168–173, 182, 188
Moral panic, 95
Moral rules, 145, 153
Moral uncertainty, 169
Movement, 1, 7, 14, 33, 38–40, 47, 49, 51, 53, 56, 61, 63, 79, 93, 96, 98, 99, 112, 117–120, 123, 124, 130, 131, 143, 145, 159, 161, 167, 171, 185
Multiculturalism, 96
Multisensory communication/gestures, 30, 32, 50, 51, 79, 98, 101, 132
Muslim, 89, 93, 96
Mutual vibration, 82

N
Nao robot, 127
National recommendations, 18
Natural element/environment/object, 82, 86–88, 102, 129, 130
Netherlands, 63
Neurological disorder, 35
Neuroscience, 15
Neutral body zone, 96
Neutral touch, 20
Newborn, 15, 16, 72, 78, 190
New Zealand, 94
Non-contact culture, 80, 95, 97
Non-human, 3, 33, 79, 85, 86, 89, 90, 122, 123, 125, 154
Non-maleficence, 146, 147
Non-procedural touch, 31
Non-verbal, 43, 48, 62, 80, 83, 84, 98–100
Normative ethics, 18, 19, 145–148, 153, 182, 189
Normative guidelines, 19, 145, 146
Normative theories, 146
Normativity, 12, 18, 19, 55, 145–148, 153, 182, 189
Norwegian, 100
No-touch policy, 94, 95, 164, 184
No touch zone, 11, 35
Nurse education, 83
Nursery school, 40, 43, 48, 94, 150
Nursing home, 35, 88, 127, 129, 163, 168, 170
Nursing science/scientist, 9, 29, 31, 43, 46, 128

O
Occupational therapist/therapy, 31, 38, 39
Oken, Lorenz, 89
Older adult, 38, 43, 83, 88, 127, 128, 131, 164
Older person, 78, 151, 166
Olfactory sensation, 50, 153
Operating theatre, 9, 112, 121
Ophthalmic, 31
Organic prosthesis or implant, 124
Organisational body, 55
Organisational culture/policy, 55, 56, 90, 189
Organisational process, 109, 110
Oxytocin, 15, 16, 189

P
Paediatric, 76
Pain, 8, 15–17, 37, 41, 42, 44, 75, 76, 92, 117, 120, 121, 123, 125, 128, 138, 151, 161
Palliative care, 3, 16, 43, 44, 54, 151, 159

Palpation, 41, 122
Palumbo, Rocco, 109, 110, 113
Parasympathetic nervous system, 15, 16, 189
Parihug, 131
Paro seal, 127
Participatory touch, 31
Paterson, Mark, 10, 11, 14, 47, 110, 126, 133, 134
Pedagogical tact/touch/skill, 31, 94, 149
Peripheral blood circulation, 41
Personal assistant, 38
Personality, 16, 32, 52, 54, 58, 63, 74, 78, 96
Personal space, 7, 9, 36, 62, 98, 100, 170
Personal trainer, 40, 54
Personal zone, 79, 185
Person-centred organisational culture, 55
Pets, 87, 88, 127
Phantom-like presence, 134
Pharmacy, 126, 138
Phenomenology, 23, 107, 112, 117–119, 129
Philosopher, philosophy, 23, 91, 112, 119, 122, 128, 143, 145, 148, 152, 153, 155, 156, 159
Phone, 108–110, 112, 114–116, 119, 125, 132, 157
Phronesis, 148–150, 188
Physical distance, 5, 86, 132, 185
Physical education, 2, 38, 95
Physical punishment, 44, 75
Physiology, 107, 134, 189
Physiotherapist/physiotherapy, 8, 20, 21, 31, 38, 39, 41, 45, 53, 77, 88, 159, 187
Pilates instruction, 40
Police officer, 2, 3, 5, 9, 10, 19, 41, 46, 57, 60, 151
Practical know-how, 149, 150
Practical wisdom, 22, 148, 188
Prejudice, 90, 156
Premature babies, 15
Pre-theoretical, 152, 153
Prima facie, 63
Primary attachment figure, 73
Primary school, 158, 163
Primate, 13–15
Private self, 60, 61
Problem-solving strategies, 117
Procedural touch, 22, 29, 31, 36–38, 48, 64, 181
Professional code, 61
Professional commitment, 146
Professional ethics, 2, 18, 23, 116, 122, 143, 145, 146, 149, 152, 154, 160, 170, 171, 187–189

Professional identity, 5, 11, 78, 117, 165–168, 182, 189
Professionalism, 17–19, 22, 30, 32, 40, 50, 51, 155, 168
Professional role, 17, 34, 61, 78, 158
Protective touch, 10, 46, 47, 59, 76, 149, 169
Proxemics, 79, 112–116, 185
Proximity, 14, 16, 32, 44, 61, 72, 73, 76, 78, 82, 83, 93, 113, 114, 184
Psyche, 45, 46, 49
Psychiatric
  care, 35, 63
  client, 35
  patient, 35, 50
  professional, 35
Psychoanalyst, 44, 73, 163
Psychological development, 16
Psychological studies, 54
Psychosis/psychotic, 59, 62, 98
Psychotherapy/psychotherapist, 21, 45, 46, 77, 95, 98, 162–164, 187
Public zone, 79, 185

R
Radiologist, 41
Rasmussen, Susan J., 89
Rational knowledge, 63
Reciprocity of touch, 11, 23, 32, 144, 154, 155, 168, 182
Refugee, 98
Rehabilitation, 39, 187
Reiki, 45
Relational body/skin, 11
Relief for symptoms, 162
Religion/religious, 12, 79–83, 99
Respectful touch, 46, 54
Reversibility, 129, 154
Rhythm, 37, 39, 50, 51, 53, 64, 87, 167
Robot/-tics, 3, 6, 10, 38, 107, 109, 117, 118, 122–129, 134
Role conflict, 163
Rosen therapy, 45

S
Safe space, 7, 80, 171, 188
Same-gender, 80, 81, 97
Saudi Arabia, 34, 65, 100
Sauna, 82
Scenarios of touch culture, 24, 182
School, 7, 20, 44, 54, 75, 94, 95, 114–116, 122, 129, 130, 133, 134, 150, 164, 166, 184

Scottish, 53, 86
Secondary caregiver, 73
Secure attachment style, 73, 75
Security guard/work, 2, 5, 31, 60, 92, 190
Segregation, 90
Self-esteem, 43, 55, 74, 133
Self-harm, 133
Self-reflection, 78
Self-service machine, 126
Self-sufficiency, 129
Sensation, 10, 14, 15, 36, 50, 63, 79, 108, 111, 122, 123, 125, 126, 129, 130, 134, 154, 159, 160, 174
Sensitive/sensitivity, 12, 19, 21, 22, 30, 62, 72, 83, 84, 93, 97–100, 144, 150, 155–160, 162, 168, 173, 182, 185, 187–189
Sensorimotor activity, 124
Sensory deprivation, 43
Sensory gesture, 12, 18, 51, 52, 59, 97, 99, 173
Sensory habit, 87
Sensory impairment, 38
Sensory order, 89
Service economy, 32, 116
Sexual abuse, 94, 98, 151, 164
Sexual connotation, 93
Sexual harassment, 6, 7, 94, 96, 172, 182, 184
Sexualised touch, 172
Sheltered house, 3, 61, 99
Sipman, Gerbert, 144, 149
Skill memory, 63
Skin colour, 83
Skin hunger, 133
Skin knowledge, 87, 88, 90
Skinscape, 3, 23, 72, 85–90, 99, 182, 189
Skinship, 85, 86
Smartphone, 2, 115, 116, 124
Smell, 4, 14, 59, 89, 130
Social distancing, 133, 182
Socialisation into touch, 13, 72–102
Socialisation practice, 90
Social media, 102, 108, 114, 190
Social position, 89, 97
Social robot, 126, 127
Social status, 85, 90
Social welfare, 145, 146
Social work/workers, 2–4, 6, 8, 10, 17, 20, 31, 32, 38, 83, 85, 110, 112, 117, 174
Social zone, 79, 185
Soft skills, 29, 30, 32, 63
Solidarity, 146, 160, 165
Somatechnic, 91

Spanish, 95
Spatial architecture, 90
Spatial context, 79
Special need, 77, 87, 190
Speech and communication impairment, 133
Sports professional, 40
State of becoming, 47
Stein, Edith, 159
Stereotype, 90, 91, 99, 100, 156
Stroke, stroking, 2, 20, 43, 127
Style of the flesh, 23, 30, 50, 61
Surface feeling, 58
Surgeon, 112, 121, 124–126
Surgical robot, 124–126
Sustainable ethics, 19, 23, 58, 143, 149, 163, 175, 182

T
Tablet, 112–114, 116
Tacit knowledge, 22, 63
Tactile defensiveness, 35
Tactile regime, 79
Tactile tactics, 33, 35
Tango, 47
Tanner, Luke, 55, 76
Task-centred organisational culture, 55
Task-oriented touch, 31, 38, 42, 93
Taste, 14, 89
Taxonomies of touch, 29, 31
Teacher, 3, 4, 7, 10, 17, 19, 20, 32, 38, 40, 43, 44, 48, 58, 60, 77, 83, 93–95, 112, 115, 116, 122, 127, 129, 130, 146, 149, 156, 158, 163–167, 172, 184, 187, 190
Technical equipment, 118, 120
Technical procedure, 96
Technological aid, 36, 121
Technological device, 2, 11, 23, 87, 88, 111, 117, 119, 120, 122, 130, 158, 190
Technological environment, 110, 182
Technological mediation, 119, 130
Technological tool, 23, 107, 108, 116–120, 182
Technologisation, 86
Technology-mediated touch, 6, 9, 23, 65, 95, 108–138, 182, 189
Technostress, 6, 113
Teenage/-r, 59, 95, 99, 133
Teleological ethics, 146
Telepresence, 133, 157
Therapeutic touch, 4, 11, 23, 29, 45–46, 49, 160, 162, 163, 181

Touch culture, 3, 5, 13, 23, 24, 55, 72–102, 108–110, 113, 114, 130, 131, 144, 150, 153, 155, 172, 174, 182, 183, 185, 187–189
Touch depression, 133, 183
Touch deprivation, 7, 23, 108, 131–134, 184
Touching style, 12, 13, 21, 52, 59, 63, 64, 78, 101
Touch norm, 13, 79, 81, 97, 100
Touch starvation, 132, 133
Touch-phobic, 133, 183
Traumatic experience, 61, 77
Triadic relationship, 120–124, 190
Triadic touch, 23, 107, 120–124, 138
Triple stigma, 95
Tuareg people, 89
Twigg, Julia, 8, 12

U

United Kingdom (UK), 82, 93, 94, 133
United States (US), 56, 58, 80, 81, 88, 90, 91, 94, 95
Universal principles, 18, 146, 147
Untouchable, 82, 83
Urban environment, 87
Urinary catheter, 36
Utilitarianism, 146

V

Value, 18, 22, 23, 30, 32, 54–57, 64, 74, 80, 84, 85, 101, 127, 130, 144–147, 149–151, 155, 160–163, 165–167, 169, 171, 174, 183
Value awareness, 19, 145, 149, 160–163, 182
Van Dongen, Els, 5, 8, 35, 36, 47, 52, 59, 63, 64, 83, 93
Ventilator, 117, 119
Verbal, 43, 48, 51, 59, 62, 83, 84, 89, 93, 123, 151, 168
Video call, 126

Video conference, conferencing, 131
Virtual, 113, 126, 132–134, 157, 190
Virtue, 18, 52, 76, 146, 148, 153, 158
Virtue ethics, 148
Visual, 14, 50, 53, 79, 83, 88, 91, 116, 120, 126, 130, 131, 133, 153
Visual-haptic technology, 125
Visually impaired, 48, 52, 117
Vocal/voice, 18, 50, 51, 56, 59, 60, 79, 114, 116, 124, 158, 167
Vulnerable
  body, 111
  client, 7, 46, 162, 189, 190
  state, 7, 46

W

Walking frame, 1, 39
Wellness, 2, 8, 12, 20, 102, 130
West/-ern, 14, 74, 82, 85, 87–91, 95, 96, 148, 183
Wheelchair, 39, 86, 118, 125
Women-only profession, 95
Work/-ing community, 52, 97, 101, 144, 150, 151, 166, 168, 171, 174, 187
World Health Organization (WHO), 5, 145
Wristband, 129

X

X-ray unit, 36

Y

Yoga, 40
Youth work, 60, 94
YouTube, 115

Z

Zora software, 127

Printed by Printforce, United Kingdom